FITNESS INC.
A GUIDE TO CORPORATE HEALTH AND WELLNESS PROGRAMS

Robert E. Pritchard
Gregory C. Potter

Medical Component
by
William S. Frankl, M.D.

Dow Jones-Irwin
Homewood, Illinois 60430

For
Marion L. Pritchard
and
Sodie E. Potter

This publication is designed to provide accurate and
authoritative information in regard to the subject matter
covered. It is sold with the understanding that the
publisher is not engaged in rendering legal, accounting, or
other professional service. If legal advice or other expert
assistance is required, the services of a competent
professional person should be sought.

From a Declaration of Principles jointly adopted by a Committee
of the American Bar Association and a Committee of Publishers.

Sponsoring editor: *Jeffrey Krames*
Project editor: *Gladys True*
Production manager: *Ann Cassady*
Jacket designer: *Sam Concialdi*
Compositor: *Better Graphics, Inc.*
Typeface: *11/13 Century Schoolbook*
Printer: *Book Press*

Library of Congress Cataloging-in-Publication Data
Pritchard, Robert E.
    Fitness, Inc.: a guide to corporate health and wellness programs
/ Robert E. Pritchard, Gregory C. Potter; medical component by
William S. Frankl; foreword by John B. Campbell.
        p. cm.
    ISBN 1-55623-274-8
    1. Health promotion. 2. Occupational health services.
I. Pritchard, Robert E., 1941–   . II. Frankl, William S.
III. Title.
RC969.H43P68   1990   89–17236
613—dc20   CIP

Printed in the United States of America

1 2 3 4 5 6 7 8 9 0 BP 6 5 4 3 2 1 0 9

FOREWORD

by John B. Campbell

Chairman of the Board of Mannington Mills, Inc.

What a piece of work is man!
How nobel in reason! How
infinite in facility! In form
and moving how express and admirable!
Hamlet, Prince of Denmark
Act II, Scene 2, by
William Shakespeare

The business of America is
business.
Calvin Coolidge

A healthy and fit workforce as well as the programs which promote wellness are essential to sound business management practices. Health and fitness in this context are defined broadly and
encompass a holistic perspective on the unity of spirit, mind, and
body. However, the wellness movement is founded upon more than
philosophical constructs and is driven by very real economic factors. When Calvin Coolidge aligned the interests of America with
those of business, he may have unwittingly announced an amal-
gam of the economic health of business with the physical and
mental health of the workforce. It has become increasingly evident
that benefits accrue to corporations from employees who are physically and mentally fit and who exhibit high levels of self-esteem.
This concept was recently emphasized in a Harvard Business

School bulletin announcing their decision to build a $20 million fitness center. It may be a truism to say that a company's employees are its most valuable asset; however, failure to recognize the wellness of employees will have significant future economic consequences.

The viability of corporate sponsored health and fitness services has been questioned on several fronts. A cause and effect relationship between wellness programs and economic indexes is much more difficult to establish than predicting the cost benefits of advancements in production technology. However, people are infinitely more complex than machines. This complexity as well as anticipated escalation of technology and changes in workforce demographics have motivated businesses to explore new alternatives for recruiting and maintaining employees.

Wellness programs have also been criticized as paternalistic by skeptics who view them as superfluous window dressing. Unfavorable attitudes have emanated in part from cynicism regarding the employer-employee relationship as well as a misunderstanding of program goals. A holistic fitness and wellness program enables individuals to make informed decisions about their lives thereby affording employees a sense of self-realization. Charges of paternalism fail to recognize that both employer and employee profit when a company is successful.

The promotion of health and fitness, therefore, has become increasingly important as a management tool. It is a tool which eludes easy analysis of projected cost benefits and which has been myopically criticized as manipulative. However, the philosophy behind wellness programs is not a phenomenon of the late 20th century. Common intellectual ground is shared with the classical civilization of the ancient Greeks whose tenets have become cornerstones of Western culture.

The Greek philosophers recognized a holism of spirit, mind, and body. This ideal sparked the Olympic spirit which venerated athletic champions, an athleticism not devoid of intellectual or spiritual purpose. An integrated concept of self emerged which placed no essential distinctions upon mind or body apart from the whole organism. This concept, driven by a very pragmatic survival instinct, may be analogous to the bottom line in modern business. Ancient civilizations faced severe physical challenges to provide food and shelter as well as defense against invasion. An effective structure for strong leadership was essential. Central to the success of the individual was integration of self. Socrates believed that a competent individual must be developed as a whole person. It would be rhetorical to question its validity today.

It is a central premise of this text that wellness programs contribute significantly to sound business management. If, however, documenting the cost effectiveness of these programs is difficult, research from other disciplines can provide a theoretical model which is both descriptive and predictive of benefits. Prospective medicine and employee relations represent two important perspectives from which to evaluate health and fitness programs.

Business and industry, which pays one half of the nation's health care bills, has become increasingly interested in primary prevention of disease. Prospective medicine recognizes that prevention is the most economically efficient way to deal with the diseases prevalent in modern society. Yet only five percent of health care dollars are spent on preventive measures.

There has been a dramatic change in the nature of disease and mortality from 1900 until the present. Early in the 20th century over 50 percent of deaths resulted from diseases caused by a specific virus or bacterium.

The situation now, however, is more complex. Cardiovascular disease and cancer, our modern-day plagues, account for over 65 percent of deaths. Moreover, epidemiologists stress that these diseases are linked more closely to personal habits or lifestyles than to any other single factor. Because no bacterium or virus causes these diseases, there are no magic bullets available to control and eliminate them. Finally, heart disease, cancer, and other lifestyle diseases develop over extended periods of time through a complex interaction between genetics and behavioral variables known as risk factors. Treatment is often delayed until the disease is far advanced and difficult to control.

For these reasons, diseases of lifestyle are extremely expensive to treat. Cardiovascular diseases alone account for $78 billion annually in direct and indirect costs. A single heart attack costs $60,000. Over 10 percent of gross national product is consumed annually by health care costs. From another perspective, the nation's yearly medical bill represents 28 percent of deficit dollars.

No statistic, however, can account for the human suffering and reduced quality of life experienced by the victims of disease. For them, no treatment, no financial expenditure, could be more efficacious than prevention.

The association between risk factors and modern disease is more than theoretical. Epidemiology links today's lifestyle to risk of disease and, more significantly, risk factor modification with disease prevention. Control of smoking and hypertension, two primary risk factors for cardiovascular disease, has resulted in a significant decline in the rate of heart disease over the past 25 years. Smoking has declined sharply from 50 to 30 percent of the population. Blood pressure control has also been a successful public health concern. Efforts to control blood cholesterol levels more adequately promise even greater positive change.

Wellness programs in business and industry represent an important adjunct to prospective medicine. Through awareness, education, and intervention, health and fitness programs can effect behavioral change, modify and control risk factors, and thereby significantly prevent disease. Moreover, large numbers of individuals can be reached at the worksite who would otherwise be unable to participate in such programs. There is no reason to suspect that corporate-based wellness programs cannot affect the same positive results that have been achieved by risk factor control within the general population.

What has been learned in prospective medicine, therefore, strongly reinforces the position of health and fitness within business. Support for the wellness movement is also based on evolving perspectives within employee relations.

Significant revision of mechanistic management models is a hallmark of modern business practice. More productive are holistic employee development plans that are responsive to both economic factors as well as individual physical, mental, and spiritual needs. Furthermore, anticipated changes in both production technology and work force demographics will require more divergent strategies to recruit and retain good employees. Competition for highly trained and motivated personnel as well as the need for continued employee development are both facilitated by wellness and other employee assistance programs.

Wellness programs accommodate not only changes in management philosophy and constituency of the work force, but are also ideally suited to address an unanticipated change in the way individuals perceive their work. Predictions of increased leisure time due to a shortened work week have not proved accurate. An article published in the March 1989 edition of *Psychology Today* reports that, compared to 15 years ago, leisure time has decreased 40 percent while time at work has actually increased by 15 percent.

A perception of work as more than a means to monetary reward is emerging. Self-enhancement and self-expression are at the foundation of a new work ethic that is exemplified by a drive to perform at one's best. Moreover, careers have for many individuals become a form of self-identity. A 1985 Gallup poll cited work-related incentives for health and fitness programs. Forty-three percent of those surveyed responded that exercise enabled them to work better and be more creative, while over 60 percent indicated that being fit made them feel more relaxed and energetic. Granted, these perceptions are highly subjective; however, they express personality traits associated with high levels of achievement and competency.

I am John B. Campbell, Chairman of the Board of Mannington Mills, Inc., manufacturer of floorcovering and ceramic tile. I represent the third generation of a large family business with 43 years of experience, and I am happy to say that the fourth generation is on the scene running the company. Regardless of my vast experience in this business world, successful businesses have one basic ingredient that makes them successful—PEOPLE! Without the right people in the right job at the right time, a company cannot be successful. It must be realized that people are the greatest hidden asset on a company's balance sheet. Accountants depreciate machinery, equipment, and buildings by several different methods, but they disregard people when determining a company's net worth. As a company grows, it will find a way to purchase more equipment and buildings by either borrowing monies or leasing, but you cannot do that with people.

If you agree with the above synopsis, then it must have occurred to you that a company must take care of its employees. How does it train, educate and prepare them for the present and future growth of the company? The older your company becomes, the greater your hidden asset of people becomes as they grow with the company. You, therefore, need to become more concerned about preserving and protecting the health and well-being of your employees for the present and the future. It was that concern and inspiration that prompted me to present my plan to our Board of Directors approximately six years ago. It began with an extremely wise discussion and ended with the building of a fitness center! Not a whim, not a perk, but a sound investment in the future of our company and of our employees.

The fitness center became a reality. It took careful planning and investing to come up with the right facilities for both indoor and outdoor requirements. As a result, very few mistakes were made. Our Board of Directors came to one very sound conclusion regarding return on capital. We feel our fitness center can prolong the life of every employee for many years, and give each employee great inspiration in the workplace and in the personal life and well-being of that individual. That satisfaction and peace of mind is a wonderful return on our investment.

INTRODUCTION

One employee said she likes
herself better since she's lost
weight. Another told us how
important exercise at the fitness
center is to her because it is her
private time to do something good
for herself. That's the kind of
impact we want to have on
employees' lives.
Burroughs Wellcome Co.
(From Chapter 5, Appendix A
of this book.)

Examining the rapid growth and evolution of the fitness/wellness movement has proven to be a most challenging and rewarding task. When we started this project, we weren't sure if the numerous corporate exercise, fitness, and various wellness programs were really "serious business" or part of a paternalistic managerial effort to keep employees happy. Then, we visited fitness centers and interviewed CEOs, vice presidents for human resources, compensation managers, fitness center managers, and members of the medical community.

We studied the whole corporate fitness/wellness movement from its beginning. What we discovered surprised us. *We found that enlightened managers recognize that people who are healthy and physically fit tend to be more productive, happier on and off the job, miss less time from the workplace, and deal more effectively with stress on and off the job! Furthermore, physically and mentally fit employees help reduce company medical insurance payments—no small consideration for many firms.* For all these reasons, many companies have established and are continuing to establish corporate fitness and wellness programs.

As we continued our research, we realized that corporate fitness and wellness programs were contributing, in both very obvious and subtle ways, to the restoration of those communal, integrative kinds of experiences that are so sorely needed in our social and work lives. By treating people holistically—as physical, mental, and spiritual beings—the many different programs we studied are helping to build positive attitudes toward self, society, and the workplace. From this perspective, *the real value of fitness and wellness programs lies in the "recreational" possibilities that these programs offer for helping people to realize their physical, social, and intellectual potential.* And by "re-creational," we mean rebuilding, restoration, not simply "leisure." Many of the corporate fitness/wellness profiles contained in Section II of this book speak directly to helping employees realize their potential in each of these areas.

Naturally, we know this idealized view must be tempered by the hard realities of today's business world. Several of the executives we interviewed spoke discouragingly of employee commitment to a profession or career, rather than to company. But the undeniable fact remains that if Corporate America is to successfully compete within the international marketplace, it must have employee commitment and dedication.

When so many good people have been subjected to the fallout resulting from merger mania and the decreasing need for middle management, it is perhaps hard to speak convincingly of "recreational possibilities" in the corporate workplace. Yet, the movement toward a caring management philosophy that we witnessed in many companies, which is particularly exemplified by the fitness/wellness movement, suggests that many companies are recommitting themselves to the long-term welfare of their employees.

In the past two tumultuous decades, we have learned to adapt to an uncertain world—a world that offers enormously exciting possibilities for social development and constructive change. As Tom Peters expresses it, business will have to learn to "thrive on chaos" if it is to succeed. In a very real sense, this means that business will have to be *fit*—fit enough to cope with stress, fit enough to adapt to dislocations, fit enough to maintain vision and commitment in an uncertain world.

Developing this corporate fitness does not involve some new, radical model of organizational behavior. On the contrary, *a fit organization is one that provides an environment that reflects a preeminent concern for people's health and sense of well-being—and the health and well-being of their families.* It simply makes good business sense to pay attention to the important personal and social concerns that affect today's worker.

Most readers want to know what quality fitness/wellness programs are all about—from fitness centers to corporate employee assistance programs. We examined numerous programs and spent days visiting sites and discussing programs with our tape recorders running. Based on our interviews and observations, we are able to provide a detailed profile of the wellness/fitness movement, indicating those characteristics which are most important to employees and employers. Moreover, in Section II of the book, we have included over 50 corporate fitness/wellness program profiles. These provide specific information detailing what companies, both large and small, are currently doing, as well as their underlying philosophies toward fitness and wellness. They warrant your careful attention.

Of course, the foundation for fitness and wellness programs lies primarily in the fields of sports and cardiac medicine. We were most fortunate to be able to interview William S. Frankl, M.D., Vischer Professor and Chairman, Department of Medicine, and Director of the Likoff Cardiovascular Institute and Division of Cardiology at Hahnemann University. He provided us with an extraordinarily rich medical basis for the fitness/well programs, while at the same time dispelling many media-popularized myths about exercise and diet. Anyone interested in personal fitness (or cardiac care) will find Section III, the Medical Aspects of Fitness/Wellness Programs, to be most informative reading.

The fitness/wellness movement in Corporate America is an important story. It is a story of American industry becoming stronger, of people living longer, and employees enjoying a more productive work experience. It is a story that speaks to a very promising future.

Robert E. Pritchard
Gregory C. Potter

ACKNOWLEDGMENTS

A project of this scope involved countless telephone calls, numerous on-site visits, and dozens of letters. We wish it were possible to thank all those people who helped directly and indirectly, but it simply would not be possible. We do most sincerely thank, however, all those fitness directors and their staffs for their extraordinarily courteous treatment and helpful suggestions. Their great enthusiasm and support for this project indeed speaks to the health and fitness of their profession!

In particular, we wish to acknowledge the contributions of:

Leo C. Beebe, Chairman and CEO, K-Tron International, Pitman, NJ.

Edward J. Bernacki, M.D., Vice President, Health, Environmental Medical and Safety, Tenneco, Inc., Houston, TX.

Dr. Robert L. Bertera, Director, Corporate Fitness, Du Pont Co., Wilmington, DE.

Warren W. Brubaker, M.D., Director, Corporate Medical Affairs, Hershey Foods Co., Hershey, PA.

Vangie Cooper, Chief, Program Support, Employment and Training Administration, Region III, U.S. Department of Labor.

Dr. Joyce H. Daniels, Assistant Professor of Psychology, Stockton State College, Pomona, NJ.

Patricia Daniels, Assistant Director, K-Tron Institute of Feeder Technology, Pitman, NJ.

Steven J. Dover, Manager, Benefits Administration, Warner-Lambert, Inc., Morris Plains, NJ.

Raymond M. Fino, Corporate Vice President—Human Resources, Warner-Lambert, Inc., Morris Plains, NJ.

Dr. James C. Gillis, President and CEO, Lifestyle Management Reports, Inc., Boston, MA.

Dr. Laurence Golding, University of Nevada.

Patricia Greebe, Corporate Communications, Burroughs Wellcome Co., Research Triangle Park, NC.

William J. Haltigan, Regional Administrator, U.S. Department of Labor, Philadelphia, PA.

Marjorie L. Hill, Director, National Information Center, Laventhol & Horwath, Philadelphia, PA.

William L. Horton, President, Fitness Systems, Los Angeles, CA.

Cheryl Howard, Manager—Corporate Health Promotion, Southwestern Bell, St. Louis, MO.

James F. Kisela, Past Vice President, Human Resources, Campbell Soup Co., Camden, NJ.

William M. Kizer, CEO, Central States Health and Life Insurance of Omaha, NE.

Frank J. LoCastro, Ed.D., Manager, Corporate Fitness, PepsiCo, Inc., Purchase, NY.

Lauve L. Metcalfe, Director of Program Development, Institute for Health and Fitness, Campbell Soup Co., Camden, NJ.

William P. Noyes, Vice President, Human Resources, Hershey Foods Co., Hershey, PA.

John Ricci, Administrator, Corporate Wellness Program, Hershey Foods Co., Hershey, PA.

Dr. David G. Romano, Lecturer, University of Pennsylvania, Philadelphia, PA.

Elizabeth Rowbotham, Wellcome Health Manager, Burroughs Wellcome Co., Research Triangle Park, NC.

Carl G. Sempier, Past President, Mannington Mills, Inc., Salem, NJ.

Dr. Barton A. Singer, Clinical Psychologist and Diplomate in Clinical Psychology, Cherry Hill, NJ.

William E. Spencer, National Director of Human Resources, Laventhol & Horwath, Philadelphia, PA.

Sandra J. Wendel, Manager, Communications, Central States Health and Life of Omaha, NE.

Robert B. Young, Manager, Take Time for Health™, Du Pont Co., Wilmington, DE.

Dr. William B. Zuti, Past Director Corporate Fitness, Pepsi-Co, Inc., Purchase, NY.

We particularly want to acknowledge and thank William S. Frankl, M.D., for the preparation of the Medical Component of this book. Dr. Frankl, Director of the Likoff Cardiovascular Institute and Chair, Department of Medicine at Hahnemann University, is recognized as one of the world's leading cardiologists. Dr. Frankl has authored three books in the field of cardiology as well as numerous articles. The Medical Component of this book represents the most up-to-date review of the medical information needed by managers today. We are most grateful to Dr. Frankl for preparing this part of the book.

We also want to thank James T. Smith, Manager, Sports Complex, Mannington Mills, Inc., Salem, N.J. Mr. Smith reviewed the entire manuscript of this book and provided very important insights and information. His input added greatly to the coverage provided.

Also, we want to acknowledge the contribution of William B. Horton, President, Fitness Systems, Los Angeles, California. Mr. Horton provided consultation throughout this project and also reviewed the entire manuscript.

We want to thank Kathleen C. Romeo, Ph.D., R.N., C.S., Assistant Professor of Nursing, Stockton State College. She reviewed the entire manuscript and offered many constructive ideas.

We also owe a very special note of thanks to our editor, Jeffrey Krames, Dow Jones-Irwin. Without his enthusiasm and encouragement, this project would not have been possible. Finally, we want to acknowledge the untiring help of Ms. Sandra Wilde, Savitz Library, Glassboro State College, for her research assistance.

R.E.P.
G.C.P.

CONTENTS

SECTION III
THE MEDICAL ASPECTS OF FITNESS/WELLNESS
PROGRAMS BY WILLIAM S. FRANKL, M.D. 323

SECTION 1

THE FITNESS AND WELLNESS MOVEMENT: PROMISE AND CHALLENGE

Managers need to understand the value of corporate fitness/wellness programs for their employees, their companies, and themselves. This section provides the information managers need to assess the organizational value and cost-effectiveness of these programs. In addition, this section provides a management perspective on stress in the workplace.

CHAPTER 1

THE NEW CORPORATE MIND/BODY PARTNERSHIP

Nations have passed away and left
no traces, and history gives the
naked source of it. One single,
simple reason in all cases—they
fell because their people were not
fit.
Rudyard Kipling

During the past several years, hundreds of companies worldwide
have developed physical fitness programs for their employees.
Many have constructed fitness centers equipped with extensive
exercise equipment, aerobic dance areas, tracks, and even swimming pools. In addition to very elaborate physical facilities, full-time professional staff are available to provide a wide range of
instructional services. Fitness programs have increasingly been
integrated with employee assistance programs (EAPs) and pre-existing medical services to provide comprehensive fitness/
wellness programs that not only help employees keep in good
physical condition, but also help them cope with such problems
as substance abuse, weight and diet control, smoking cessation,
and stress.

As we studied the fitness movement, we became aware that it
represents a significant new corporate attitude toward employees.
Employees were once viewed in the old "scientific management"
model as replaceable "units" in some systems-model of production.
Now, instead, the fitness/wellness movement implies that employees are fundamentally physical, mental, and spiritual beings
whose attitudes, values, and feelings affect their overall sense of
well-being and that of the company as well.

We then asked ourselves if the fitness/wellness movement
truly is representative of a pervasive change in management

philosophy away from a strictly "bottom-line", hard economic approach, toward a more genuinely caring, humanistic approach. Or, can the many excellent programs we saw in action be more narrowly viewed within management philosophy and practice—maybe as just another relatively low-cost perk or perhaps simply as recreation?

From our studies, we believe that the fitness/wellness movement is in a significant evolutionary phase. From its earlier roots as a means of containing health care costs, the fitness/wellness industry now is moving toward becoming an integral part of an organizational development plan designed to help employees cope with a highly stressful, highly competitive, and volatile international business environment. Ironically, the evolution of fitness/wellness programs today toward a more humanistic, caring approach is a direct consequence of three important economic factors. Based on our interviews with executives and fitness managers, these factors, in their order of importance, are as follows:

1. *Changes in the labor force which will dramatically reduce the supply of available skilled labor.* We have concluded that the changes in the composition and size of the labor force, which are already being felt, will likely have the greatest single impact on the fitness/wellness movement during the next 10 to 15 years. We detail some of those changes that particularly affect the fitness/wellness movement later in this chapter.

2. *Recognition of the bottom-line health benefits that can be derived from employees who are healthy, physically fit, and who have positive self-images.* Although some scholars have criticized the statistical and methodological rigor of some of the major health promotion studies in the corporate workplace, widespread consensus nonetheless exists on the major components relating to good health (good nutrition, avoidance of substance abuse, and appropriate levels and kinds of exercise). Many managers are positively convinced that significant bottom-line improvements can result from helping employees to stay fit, healthy, and in good spirits. Nearly all of the corporate fitness/wellness profiles contained in Section II of this book speak to the high value that Corporate America places on good health programs.

3. *Recognition of the bottom-line attitudinal and moti-*

vational benefits which can be produced by treating employees in a caring and humane manner. Again, rigorous academic support for the proposition that fitness/wellness programs contribute in a principal way to enhanced employee motivation and morale may not be forthcoming for some time (the fitness/wellness movement is still young and benefits cannot be realized in a short-term perspective). But numerous corporate executives we interviewed expressed the conviction that caring companies are more profitable, and especially so in the long run. Many autocratic managers would disagree. A debate, however, is hardly necessary. *Barring an economic catastrophe during the next few years, the shortage of skilled labor will shrink to the point where, as a practical matter, managers will need to treat their employees well in order to retain them.*

Over the years, many books have been written extolling the virtues of caring for employees as whole people. As William Walton, cofounder of Holiday Inns, for example, remarked so poignantly in his book, *The New Bottom Line,* "In the business world . . . it is the mandate and mission of an excellent manager to create conditions in the workplace where people will be energized and encouraged to stretch toward the greatest self-realization."[1]

We couldn't agree more! With the upcoming labor shortage, it will be essential to get 100 + percent out of people in order to survive in the international marketplace.

The fact is that *Corporate America faces a real problem.* Throughout the 80s we witnessed a tremendous restructuring of business. Merger mania may have produced some operating efficiencies (or inefficiencies), but it also resulted in the dislocation of hundreds of thousands of employees—good people who worked hard and were committed to their employers, but who were nevertheless abandoned by those employers, frequently with very short notice.

Similarly, the elimination of layers of middle management within many companies has added to corporate efficiencies but has taken a tremendous human toll in the form of layoffs, early retirements, and the lack of potential upward job growth for remaining employees. These have contributed to the destruction of that very important bond which heretofore had existed between most employers and employees. William P. Noyes, Vice President,

Human Resources, Hershey Foods Company,[2] states the situation faced by Corporate America very succinctly:

> Attitude surveys show that employees are feeling less caring about their companies. People planned to work for the same company until retirement. They felt a commitment to it and thought it had a commitment to them. In the last few years, however, employees have witnessed corporate takeovers and the elimination of jobs. Many companies are coming across as not caring in general. Now employees are saying that they care about themselves and their professions first.
>
> Companies now realize that the employee always must be kept in mind. A company, after all, is only as good as its employees. What makes one company better than another is not simply technology. Sure, margins may be better and a company may be more competitive in the short run, but this is short-term thinking. If you have an employee committed to trying to help you make the company more productive, and, in effect, to do a job with three people where four may have done it before—that makes the difference between an excellent company and an average company.

FINANCIAL REALITIES AND CARING MANAGEMENT

> In spite of the cost of
> living, it's still popular.
> *Kathleen Norris*

How does Mr. Noyes' statement relate to the financial realities facing Corporate America? Examine the financial reality first. Companies are bottom-line driven. They are measured every 90 days by the results of their quarterly earnings reports. Their very existence depends on their financial performance. If earnings or anticipated earnings decrease, shareholders abandon the stock without hesitation, thereby precipitating a decline in the market price. Shareholders are fickle. With rare exception, they have no vested interest in the companies they own. Their interest is purely financial and very frequently short term. Consequently, management is driven to produce profits. If it does not, it will be replaced. If it does, it will be rewarded, often very handsomely.

Mr. Noyes, along with other enlightened managers, recognizes that many companies, which are increasingly under the gun to be profitable, have seriously compromised or destroyed altogether the employee trust now desperately needed to compete effectively. Companies now are beginning to recognize that to regain employee trust, management must treat their employees in a caring manner.

We agree with Mr. Noyes and those many other managers we interviewed that a more humanistic approach toward employees is needed. The issue does not center on some "spiritual revolution" taking place within the management community. Managers, for the most part, are pragmatists and of necessity must be concerned with goals and end results. In fact, given the growth of worldwide trade and worldwide financial markets, business is probably more bottom-line oriented today than at any time in the past.

No "free lunch" for humanistic approaches exists any more than there is a "free lunch" for anything. Even the most benevolent intentions for improving employee well-being must be reconciled with the costs of implementation and administration. Managers will become more caring and will take a real interest in all aspects of employee fitness/wellness because they ultimately depend upon highly productive, motivated employees— employees who are committed to their work and who are prepared to accept a level of stress and uncertainty in their careers and jobs.

Raymond Fino, Vice President, Human Resources, Warner-Lambert,[3] expresses the interconnection between the bottom line and establishing a fitness center for employees this way:

> About 50 percent of the decision to establish a fitness/wellness program at Warner-Lambert was based on the financial benefits. Make no mistake about it, we are here to return wealth to the shareholders. That is the only reason we exist. To the extent that the shareholder is getting his money's worth, we are able to provide opportunities to our employees.
>
> If I didn't have the confidence that we were getting more out of our fitness center than we are putting in, I think it would have been a much more difficult proposition for us to sell.

Frank J. LoCastro, Ed.D., Manager of Corporate Fitness at PepsiCo, Inc.,[4] drives home the point about the necessity for caring for employees in a tight labor market:

Since the beginning of the health and fitness movement in this country, PepsiCo has provided its employees with state-of-the-art health and fitness programming.

The philosophy behind PepsiCo's ongoing wellness commitment to its employees is based not on the cost effectiveness of these programs and how they affect the bottom line, but rather on the premise that these programs are an important and necessary employee benefit and should be made available to any employee who wishes to participate.

Does this mean that if labor markets were to expand and more qualified people were to become available, Corporate America's attitude toward employees would revert to more traditional, less humanistic values and that fitness/wellness programs would be terminated? Probably not! The overwhelming evidence today indicates that employers do get higher productivity from employees who are "treated right" by their employers and from employees who are both mentally and physically fit and who have high levels of self-esteem.

The management community has already begun to recognize that employees who lack self-esteem and who do not feel good about themselves have little, if any, motivation to improve their health. Consequently, they are likely to exhibit increased absenteeism, have more frequent need of counseling or other medical services, and, taken in the aggregate, contribute to lowered levels of productivity and quality control. Poor health is clearly a poor example, if not an affront, to those who do take care of themselves. Indeed, the issues surrounding the rights of the nonsmoker speak to a growing public awareness of good health and the sense that it is one's social responsibility to promote good health, whether in the home, at school, or in the workplace.

Most managers know that if they take the time, they can help to build employee self-esteem by praise, pats on the back, or involving employees with their work. Building employee self-esteem will inculcate a desire on the part of employees to take better care of themselves, be healthier, have lower absenteeism, and exhibit higher productivity.

In short, management is recognizing that caring about employees' physical and mental health makes real bottom-line sense. This message has already gained a foothold and will make inroads as the supply of labor continues to contract. Over the next decade, these facts likely will be integrated into existing organizational behavior models. Moreover, managers will be trained in the bottom-line aspects of fitness/wellness programs.

Leo C. Beebe, Chairman and CEO of K-Tron International,[5] describes the bottom-line importance of physically fit and alert employees this way:

> In all organizations, it is the people who make the difference. Our products and services are not what makes us competitive. The equipment can sit there unused (at the customer's place of business), if we don't have the people who know how to counsel with the customer, relate to the customer and communicate with the customer. Our customers are people and relate best to physically fit, alert people.

There is no question that management philosophy changes to meet the conditions of the day. Today, those conditions include a very strong emphasis on performance and a shortage of qualified labor. Accordingly, managers who expect to attract and retain qualified help will have to learn to treat their people right and help them keep healthy and fit. That is the reality facing managers.

FINANCIAL JUSTIFICATION FOR PHYSICAL FITNESS FACILITIES AND PROGRAMS

> Nothing ruins a class reunion like
> a fellow who has managed to stay
> young-looking and get rich at the
> same time.
> *Indianapolis Star*

During our interviews, we spoke with managers who related stories about their CEO or some other senior-level executive who, after having had a heart attack or bypass surgery, became involved with his or her own physical fitness and then decided that the company should build a fitness center for employees. How do these stories stand up against the harsh financial realities described earlier?

A fitness facility is a capital investment. The dollars to build and equip a fitness center must come from somewhere. That "somewhere," of course, is the same source for all other projects, namely, the company's capital budget. All proposed projects compete for scarce dollars. Similarly, the dollars to operate a fitness program and meet all other expenses (including medical insurance for employees and absenteeism) must come out of operating budgets.

Which proposed projects and programs are approved? Generally speaking, those judged most likely to generate the greatest after-tax cash flow (and profit) per dollar of cost over their projected lives. Capital expenditures, including those for fitness centers as well as programmatic expenditures, are based on cold, hard, cash flow and profit projections. Existing fitness centers were not built on someone's whim. They were constructed and continue to operate because they have passed and continue to pass the rigorous analysis inherent in the ongoing capital budgeting process.

These rigorous procedures have posed, and will continue to pose, problems for many proponents of fitness/wellness programs. Numerous studies have been undertaken with the goal of substantiating the financial value of fitness centers and of fitness/wellness programs. Although many of these studies appear to provide strong, empirical evidence for the benefits of fitness/wellness programs in the workplace, a number of managers we interviewed remain skeptical about such "hard data" studies. They believe that it is very difficult to demonstrate, for example, the impact of implementing a smoking cessation and stress reduction program or constructing a fitness center, and especially so in the short run. (See Chapter 2 for more information on justifying fitness/wellness programs.)

Yet, we know that people who don't smoke are healthier than people who do. We also know that people who smoke and have other self-abusing habits tend to focus on their habits. They seek to find ways to serve the "nicotine god." Similarly, people who are not physically fit tend to feel sick or tired more often than their fit counterparts. Those who are less fit tend to focus more on how they feel rather than on the job at hand. This decreases their productivity—we all know that—yet we can't quantify it very readily. We also know that people who are well don't want to work around people who are sick. People who are habitually ill in a work setting distract and annoy those who are well and, consequently, decrease the well employees' productivity. Again, this "truth" is not readily quantifiable.

The situation faced by fitness proponents is analogous to that faced by companies deciding to build new offices or plants. Do companies build aesthetically pleasing, open, hospitable buildings, or do they simply throw up inexpensive Quonset huts? Years ago many "functional" facilities were constructed that now are regarded as horrible monuments to "low-cost bidding." Most companies recognize that the appearance of facilities has an impact on employee morale and that there is a positive relationship between a good physical work environment and employee productivity, even though it is very difficult to quantify some aspects of that relationship. If companies did not accept this relationship, we would all be working in those Quonset huts.

We similarly would argue that fitness/wellness programs do provide significant bottom-line returns even though it may be many years before conclusive longitudinal studies provide validation. Raymond Fino, Vice President, Human Resources, Warner-Lambert[6] summed it up this way:

> A study to measure the cost effectiveness of our fitness program would cost in the range of $100,000. We did a lot of research before we went into it. We believe that the program is financially viable and that we don't need to measure it. It relieves stress and results in higher productivity and reduced overall health care costs for those who participate.
>
> There is certainly more than a one-to-one return per dollar of investment to bottom-line productivity from fitness centers. I can argue for the fitness centers to our shareholders in terms of long-term productivity. For every dollar we spend, we are getting back that plus some factor as a result of reduced medical premiums, higher productivity, and higher morale.

Enlightened managers recognize the value of fitness/wellness programs. *The key question managers now should address is not the financial viability of fitness/wellness programs, but rather the delivery systems for those programs.* For example, does a company build its own fitness facility, provide memberships for employees at a local YMCA or health club, or encourage employees to become fit in some other program? Similarly, does a company use in-house personnel or contract with outside vendors? As noted in Section II, there are many different approaches. Compaq Computer Corporation, for example, channels many of its activities through a unique association with a YMCA adjacent to the Compaq campus.

In the following section we highlight the principal trends taking place in the labor market that will impact upon all employee service programs, including fitness/wellness programs. Central to all of these trends is the basic fact that employers will have to provide more non-wage benefits, in addition to the traditional wage and benefits packages, if they expect to compete successfully in the labor market of the 21st century.

In the final section of this chapter, we summarize the specific implications for management which will result from dramatic changes in the labor markets.

THE CHANGING LABOR MARKETS

The squeaking wheel doesn't
always get the grease.
Sometimes it gets replaced.
Vic Gold

Our specific interest is how the labor markets will be changing between now and the year 2000. We believe this information is crucial, since changes in the labor markets clearly affect management's attitude toward labor, especially if the markets are not expanding as rapidly as demand for labor, which is exactly what is and will continue to happen for the next 10 to 15 years.

A number of very significant demographic and economic changes are taking place in the United States that will have a major impact on the work force. The demographic changes result primarily from the end of the baby boom and the decrease in the number of young people who will be entering the labor force between now and the year 2000. Furthermore, the labor participation rate, which has been increasing for years primarily as a result of more women entering the labor force, will continue to increase but at a considerably slower rate.

In addition, we note three other important changes. The first involves the demographics of birthrates. Hispanics and blacks have higher birth rates than whites so there will be proportionately more minorities entering the labor force. Many of these minority entrants will come from nonworking welfare families and will need to be assimilated into the labor force. In particular, many will have to be convinced that it is in their best financial and social interests to work rather than to be on welfare.

Second, there will continue to be substantial immigration, both legal and illegal. Projections from the U.S. Department of Labor indicate that both the Hispanic and Asian populations likely will double—to 30 and 10 million, respectively—by the year 2000. These groups will represent a wide variety of educational and job-skill levels.

Finally, while the trend of increasing participation of females in the work force will slow, relatively more women than men will be entering the work force.

Between now and the year 2000, minorities, immigrants, and women will make up about 85 percent of the additions to the work force; white males will make up only about 15 percent. Traditionally, these three emerging employment groups have been disadvantaged in having less education and skills training than their white male counterparts.

A major problem facing employers will be the inability of many workers to be fully productive when hired because of a lack of basic education and/or skills training. Many employers will have to plan for in-house basic education (including literacy, in some cases) and skills training programs. The high school dropout rate in major industrial cities ranges around 40–50%. Consequently, employers will be forced to either hire less-skilled workers or compete for a limited number of skilled workers in a very tight labor market.

Although the health status of Americans has improved greatly over recent decades, health resources are not uniformly available to all groups in society. Many poorer households are not covered by health insurance programs. These households, which typically are represented by a greater proportion of part-time and temporary workers, tend to evidence more health problems and therefore constitute a potential wellness problem for employers.

As labor shortages intensify, more employers will make accommodations in their work force practices to attract women. Probably one of the most important accommodations will be the need for employers to become more flexible in their approach to work assignments—to be more creative so that people can work varying hours (flex-time) or work in part-time positions. Cottage industries probably will continue to grow, although some studies indicate that the lack of socialization in a home-based work context may raise problems for the employer.

Providing assistance in child care will become very important. More and more, we see single-parent families, rather than the traditional family with a husband and a wife. The proportion of children being brought up in single-parent families is significantly greater than 50 percent. In addition, two-worker families are becoming the norm. In the next decade, employers who need a top-quality workforce will have to make accommodations to meet the needs of both single and married parents.

Changes in technology, such as robotics, will continue to decrease the number of lower-skilled production jobs but, at the same time, will require workers with higher levels of education and training. Increasing use of high technology equipment has opened whole new fields in the production and maintenance of machines.

Within the production arena, companies will be faced with a new dimension when making capital budgeting decisions. Historically, the decision to substitute technology and equipment for labor was based on the premise that companies could hire qualified labor to operate the proposed equipment. This assumption no longer may be correct. A senior executive at a large food manufacturing company indicated that management was considering more low-tech rather than high-tech facilities as a consequence of the expected shortage of qualified, skilled labor.

The upcoming shortage in labor may also result in some

very positive side effects. Executives we interviewed discussed three:

1. *A continuing increase in employment with a concurrent decrease in unemployment.* This will result in higher federal and state income tax revenues and reduced unemployment payments.

2. *A breaking away from the generation-after-generation welfare society that has developed, especially within the inner city.* The economics are right for a reduction in the number of welfare recipients, as companies hire these people, train them, and provide the needed day care. Getting people off the welfare rolls obviously has positive implications with respect to limiting future increases in government spending.

3. *A decrease in racial and other forms of discrimination.* Historically, discrimination has resulted largely from economic deprivations. Job protection by unions, for example, was based on the premise that the number of jobs was limited. The contraction in the available supply of labor should help to reduce job discrimination.

IMPLICATIONS FOR MANAGEMENT

The executive exists to make
sensible exceptions to general
rules.
Etling E. Morison

Based on our interviews with executives and managers, we anticipate that a number of important changes will occur in management's accommodations to employees and in employee benefits. These are described below.

Management Accommodations to Employees

1. *Employers will have to expand their fitness/wellness programs* to meet the needs of a more fitness-conscious recruit as well as of an aging work force. Although the traditional wage-benefits package will remain a key factor in recruitment and retention, physical fitness programs will be used increasingly as tools for recruitment and retention.

2. *Employers will have to offer flexible hours, part-time positions, and job sharing* to meet the needs of employable retirees as well as the many women (and an increasing number of men) who do not desire full-time employment.

3. *Employers will be forced to hire less-qualified workers* (or pay a very high price for more skilled workers). Consequently, skills training and education programs for these new employees will be needed, as well as programs encouraging motivation and productive work skills.

4. *Employers will have to provide for employees' child care.*

5. *Employers will have to provide for extensive and ongoing management training* in employee stress reduction, communications, and employee motivation.

Employee Benefits

1. *Employers will have to recognize that some components of the traditional benefits package, such as life insurance, health insurance, and pensions, will become less important* to many new employees and especially the young professional employees. Why? Simply because one has to die to benefit from life insurance or be sick to benefit from medical insurance. Young professionals want benefits they can use now, such as a fitness center, to stay in shape.

2. *Employers will have to enhance their employee assistance programs,* especially those dealing with emotional and stress counseling and substance abuse. Employee stress and stress-related illnesses are becoming an increasingly serious and expensive problem for management.

3. *Employers will have to adjust insurance co-payments and deductibles to reflect individual fitness/wellness.* Employer and employee will assume a partnership in health promotion, with incentives offered to employees who take care of themselves.

We believe, therefore, that employers will have to take a much more *holistic approach* toward employee fitness/wellness as a direct consequence of the changes which are emerging within the economy and the labor markets.

WHAT'S AHEAD

Earlier in this chapter we indicated that the validity of the data obtained from studies designed to demonstrate the cost-effectiveness of fitness/wellness programs has been questioned to some degree. Nonetheless, we argue that the data gathered from such organizations as Johnson & Johnson, Control Data, and others warrants the attention of anyone seriously interested in the fitness/wellness movement. In Chapter 2, we summarize and describe some of the important studies that have been used to justify fitness/wellness programs.

ENDNOTES

1. William B. Walton, with Dr. Mel Lorentzen, *The New Bottom Line: People and Loyalty in Business* (San Francisco: Harper & Row, 1986), p. 23.
2. Interview with William P. Noyes.
3. Interview with Raymond M. Fino.
4. Interview with Frank J. LoCastro
5. Interview with Leo C. Beebe.
6. Interview with Raymond M. Fino.

CHAPTER 2

THE BOTTOM-LINE VALUE OF FITNESS/WELLNESS PROGRAMS

People who don't know if they
are coming or going are
usually in the biggest hurry
to get there.

In Chapter 1 we said that the philosophy of fitness/wellness programs is intuitively appealing—people who are physically fit and take care of themselves by not smoking, not drinking excessively, taking steps to minimize stress, and using seat belts will have lower absenteeism, incur fewer medical bills, and be more productive than their less-healthy contemporaries. Numerous studies have been conducted to quantify these relationships and to demonstrate the savings in health-related costs for those companies with fitness/wellness programs.

The underlying logic that a healthy, fit individual will be more productive than his or her out-of-shape counterpart is indeed very compelling—compelling to the point that many companies already have established, and others are establishing, employee exercise and wellness programs and constructing fitness centers.

Based on our interviews with managers, we conclude that the fitness/wellness train left the station long ago and is gaining momentum rapidly. Many companies are convinced that fitness/wellness programs return much more than the relatively modest costs involved in building and operating facilities and/or establishing exercise and wellness programs. Frequently, managers told us that "our company does not need to spend thousands of dollars on studies to show that we get back at least what we spent on our fitness center (or program), and probably a lot more in terms of improved productivity and reduced absenteeism."

LOOKING FOR "HARD" DATA

> The trouble with advice is that
> you seldom know whether it is good
> or bad until you no longer need
> it.

The first step in trying to justify any capital or programmatic expenditure, such as a fitness/wellness program—whether facilities are involved or not—requires financial data: What are the costs? What are the benefits and when will each be incurred? The answers to these questions are generally not available in-house since few companies have had much experience in the management and tracking of fitness/wellness programs.

To demonstrate the decision-making process, consider a company evaluating the use of a "Wear Your Seat Belt" program. The company probably would contact one or more vendors of such programs. Based on the vendors' estimates of the increase in the number of employee and family members who will always use their seat belts after completing the program, and on the vendors' estimates of the savings to the company resulting from greater seat belt usage, management would make a "go" or "no go" decision.

Of course, management would have no way of knowing if the choice in favor of the "go" decision was, in fact, the correct one until follow-up studies over a period of years were completed. These follow-up studies would be designed to determine how many more employees and family members actually became seat belt wearers and, of those additional seat belt wearers, how many actually continued to wear their belts for some period of time. The goal of these follow-up studies would be to determine the cost savings to the company resulting from the additional employees using seat belts.

In the interim, of course, many of these employees may have left the company and contacting them could prove difficult and expensive. Also, auto manufacturers may have since designed an "automatic" seat belt or installed inflatable air bags which would render the study moot. The simple fact is that in many cases the cost of undertaking follow-up studies could be many times greater than the cost of the program and the results of the studies could prove to have little, if any, relevance to future decisions regarding other fitness/wellness programs.

Consider a second example: smoking cessation programs. Members of the medical community indicate that, depending on how long and how much a person has smoked, it may take upwards of 10 to 15 years (after the person stops smoking) before the chances of that person contracting lung cancer, cardiovascular disease, or other smoking-related disease is reduced to the same level as it is for a person who has never smoked. Consequently, a major potential benefit of having a smoking cessation program (saving the cost of medical bills associated with lung cancer, for example) may be many years down the road.

Certainly, however, the reformed smoker may be healthier (have fewer colds and better aerobic capacity) and therefore exhibit a lower rate of absenteeism. Given the relatively low cost of a smoking cessation program, even these immediate benefits may more than justify the cost of sponsoring the program.

When undertaking a cost-benefit analysis, it is most important to realize that those potential "high dollar" cost savings associated with a program like smoking cessation are not likely to be enjoyed until some time in the future, if at all! In fact, they may never be realized if, for instance, an employee who happens to contract a costly disease is no longer covered by the company's insurance plan or if a cure for the disease is discovered. In addition, the cost of the treatment may escalate rapidly as a result of inflation or decrease appreciably as a result of new methods of treatments. Consequently, attempts to estimate medical cost savings that might be realized in 15 to 20 years from actions taken today represent speculation at best. *Attempting to include potential distant future benefits (or costs) of a smoking cessation (or similar) program in a cost-benefit analysis makes little sense from the viewpoint of financial analysis.*

Based on industry practices in the field of capital budgeting, we recommend discounting heavily any expected benefits or costs attributable to fitness/wellness programs which are expected to be enjoyed or incurred beyond a five-year horizon.

> Long-range investing under rapidly changing
> conditions, especially under conditions that
> change or may change at any moment under the
> impact of new commodities and technologies,
> is like shooting at a target that is not only
> indistinct but moving and moving jerkily at
> that.
> *J. A. Schumpter,* Capitalism, Socialism, and Democracy
> *(New York: Harper & Row, 1947), p. 88.*

CAPTURING ALL THE COSTS AND BENEFITS OF A FITNESS/WELLNESS PROGRAM

In evaluating most fitness/wellness programs, certain potential costs are often overlooked. Kenneth Warner[1] notes that there may be indirect consequences to fitness/wellness programs which may result in expenditures not normally factored into a cost-benefit analysis. For example, consider the person who stops smoking and thereby increases his or her expected life-span. Assuming this person is covered by the company's pension, the company, by sponsoring a smoking cessation program, may be increasing its potential pension liability. In addition, it may also be increasing its future medical costs, since the reformed smoker is likely to incur medical costs during those "added" years of his or her life.

The overriding question is the relevance of these costs to a re-alistic cost-benefit analysis. We conclude that such costs are likely to be insignificant on a present-value basis. For example, assume an employee is 50 years old and is expected to live to age 70, re-tiring at 70 or before. Furthermore, let's assume that by changing his or her lifestyle as a result of involvement in a company fitness/wellness program, his or her life expectancy will increase by two years. In addition, let's say that the company will pay the person a pension of $15,000 per year for those two years. Applying a conservative discount rate of 8 percent, the present value of the additional two years of pension payments is less than $6,000.

Is the conservative 8 percent discount rate appropriate in this calculation? Many financial managers would argue that it is too conservative because of the very great degree of uncertainty surrounding the events that could take place during the 20-year period in question. A more realistic discount rate would be 12 percent. Applying this rate yields a present value of the two-years added pension of about $2,500. *Again, we recommend discounting heavily any expected benefits or costs attributable to fitness/wellness programs which are expected to be enjoyed or incurred beyond a five-year horizon.*

As a final note to this section on cost-benefit analysis, we point to the rather compelling evidence from the insurance industry. This industry, which probably has more statistical data on medical costs and mortality rates than most others, has a disproportionately large number of fitness/wellness programs. Maybe the insurers know something other companies are just learning.

GOVERNMENT AND MILITARY HEALTH AND WELLNESS DATA

> The first big lie: I'm from
> the government and I'm here to
> help you.

U. S. Department of Health and Human Services

From the "hard data" standpoint, the federal government recognizes that "a better understanding of the connections between diet, smoking, and other aspects of lifestyle and good health seems to have altered many American habits."[2] These behavioral changes are documented in *The 1990 Health Objectives for the Nation: A Midcourse Review*, published by the Public Health Service of the U.S. Department of Health and Human Services.

This report, prepared in 1985, examines the progress toward the realization of the health objectives that were outlined in the Surgeon General's 1979 publication of *Healthy People: The Surgeon General's Report on Health Promotion and Disease Preven-*

tion. This extensive document identified 226 health objectives and measures to improve health in 15 areas of mortality, morbidity, preventive interventions, and health-related behaviors for the target year 1990.

To help provide a sure footing for the basic substance of fitness and wellness programs, it is useful to outline the appropriate comments that appear in the *Midcourse Review*. The *Review*'s reports are noted below:

High Blood Pressure Control

Controlling high blood pressure has proven to be one of the most effective means available for reducing mortality in the adult population. Death rates from heart disease and stroke—both of which are linked causally to elevated blood pressure—continue to rank first and fourth among causes of death in the United States, according to 1984 provisional data. . . .

Smoking and Health

Cigarette smoking is recognized as the most important single preventable cause of death in our society.

Physical Fitness and Exercise

Regular physical activity can benefit a person's health in a number of ways. Established benefits include reduced risk of coronary heart disease, improved ability to maintain desired weight, reduced symptoms associated with temporary anxiety states and relief from the feelings and other symptoms associated with mild to moderate depression. In addition, people who engage in regular physical activity report that they feel better generally and have more energy.

Stress

Regarding control of stress, the report comments that "By 1990, stress identification and control should become integral components of the continuum of health services offered by organized health programs." The *Review* does not offer the same kind of clear, positive statement on stress that it does for the other categories, principally because stress control is too new an area of research. The *Review* does state, however, that knowledge of stress management and the effects of stress has expanded significantly.

Clearly, the data provided by the federal government speaks convincingly to the financial viability of fitness/wellness programs.

U. S. Navy

The U. S. Navy, in its "Fighting Fit" worksite intervention program, draws upon an organizational behavior framework integrating behavioral theories from many disciplines. The program, which targets interventions at three levels—organizational/environmental, group, and individual—includes a comprehensive program evaluation consisting of lifestyle questionnaires distributed at baseline and one year, fitness and body fat testing conducted semiannually, and the use of a matched control worksite. All active duty personnel are surveyed and tested.[3]

At the present time, complete evaluation is still pending; however, significant improvements in physical fitness testing were noted at the intervention site. The program also appears to be well-accepted by most individuals assigned to a West Coast Naval Station.[4]

THE ROLE OF THE INSURANCE INDUSTRY

> A life insurance salesman was
> standing beside a tractor
> trying to sell a policy to a
> farmer. The farmer looked
> down and said, "No, I want no
> life insurance—when I die I
> want it to be a sad day for
> everyone."

Within the private sector, the insurance industry assumes an increasingly important role in basic research on health and wellness. The American Council of Life Insurance has compiled data from 418 companies for the reporting category "Health and Wellness." Interestingly, the Council lists 16 subcategories that, taken together, give an indication of the breadth and depth of the fitness/ wellness movement:

- Periodic health exam
- Exercise fitness
- Smoking cessation
- Weight control
- Hypertension screening
- Nutrition
- Stress management
- Cardiopulmonary resuscitation
- Drug/alcohol abuse
- Heart attack risk reduction
- Cancer risk reduction
- Hypertension control
- Health risk appraisal
- Accident risk reduction
- Family planning
- Other

In the "Other" category, the Council notes that companies are increasingly reporting fitness/wellness activities in this subcategory for such important areas as AIDS education, blood drives, lunchtime health lectures and activities, and employee assistance programs.

In addition to tracking data on corporate health and wellness within the business sector, the Council participates in numerous research and development programs for companies that are interested in health promotion. One such program, for example, includes a major four-year research project to develop and evaluate self-help smoking cessation resources aimed primarily toward black workers.

INDUSTRY AND PRIVATE AGENCY DATA

Experience is knowing a lot
of things you shouldn't do.
William S. Knudsen

Numerous agencies and companies have collected data on health and wellness. A sampling of information follows.

The American Heart Association

Among the many private agencies concerned with the improvement of public health, the American Heart Association (AHA) has taken a strong position favoring the promotion of health and fitness within the business sector. Stressing "compelling economic reasons" behind the need for business to promote cardiovascular health, the AHA cites the clear evidence for the "return on investment reported by businesses that have conducted health promotion programs."[5] According to the AHA, the benefits of worksite health promotion programs include the ability of employees to work harder and to show greater motivation, which leads to improved employer/employee relations and greater productivity.[6]

The American Diabetes Association

The American Diabetes Association (ADA), recognizing that diabetes affects many aspects of one's health, has launched a nationwide "corporate wellness" program, "Working on Winning," to promote awareness not only of diabetes, but also the importance of "general good health practices" for employers and employees alike. The ADA cites "reduced medical claims, fewer doctor office visits, diminished need for acute care and treatment, less hospitalizations, and decreased absenteeism on the job" as some of the important results of educational intervention in diabetes.[7]

Provider Company Data

An additional and important research base in fitness/wellness programs can be found in the extensive studies conducted by such provider companies (companies that market fitness/wellness programs) as Control Data Corporation, Johnson & Johnson, Du Pont, and Fitness Systems. These corporations have pioneered programs covering all facets of fitness and wellness and also have conducted longitudinal studies to assess the impact of their programs on reducing health-related costs for their subscribers.

Control Data Corporation

Control Data Corporation,[8] which markets the "StayWell"™ program, maintains that the results from a recent major study "demonstrate conclusively" that

> a significant difference exists in the utilization and cost of medical care by health risk status. Generally, high-risk persons utilize more medical care than other persons and generate high claim costs.

Specifically, the study reveals that

- Employees who smoke a pack or more a day of cigarettes have medical claim costs that are 18 percent higher than those of employees who do not smoke.
- Sedentary employees have 30 percent more hospital days than those who get adequate levels of exercise.
- Seriously overweight employees are 48 percent more likely to have claims exceeding $5,000 during a one-year period than those at normal weights.

The "StayWell" database, one of the largest of its kind, includes "Health Risk Profile" results on more than 30,000 different employees. According to Control Data Corporation, data has been carefully scrutinized and found to exceed the requirements for meaningful analysis.

Johnson & Johnson

Another highly respected provider, Johnson & Johnson,[9] has developed a comprehensive and extensive evaluation system in support of its "Live for Life"™ program. In commenting on the cost-benefit projections of this program, George and Hembree[10] highlight that "'Live for Life' wellness can break even on an operating basis in year three with a payout in year five." These reporters also comment that these figures "do not include the benefits gained from improved morale, satisfaction with supervision, and organizational commitment."

Fitness Systems

Fitness Systems[11] another provider, gives this summary of several studies on the benefits of fitness/wellness programs:

In general, the studies found positive benefits in (1) reduced health care and insurance costs, (2) lowered absenteeism and turnover and (3) enhanced productivity and working effectiveness. For example, employees who participated in work site exercise programs evidenced decreased rates of absenteeism ranging from 2.5 to 8.6 days per employee per year. Annual health care expenditures for exercisers were found to be from $200 to $600 less per employee than for non-exercisers. The exercisers at one company had a turnover rate 13.5 percent below that of the non-exercising controls.

Another company which did not evaluate turnover rates specifically reported an observation of lower turnover among exercisers. The productivity of departments with exercisers at an experimental company increased three percent more than at a control company which had no exercise program. Finally, another study found that active exercisers tended to be above average job performers.

Central States Health & Life Co. of Omaha

William M. Kizer, Chairman and CEO of Central States Health & Life Co. of Omaha,[12] provided strong support for fitness/wellness programs:

> I think wellness programs send out a strong message that management cares about its people. I think that a company which does not have a program would, over a period of time, attract people who do not care about their health. A company with a healthy workforce has lower absenteeism and higher productivity. Wellness programs also improve the esprit de corps. Our turnover rate over the last five years is significantly below average for the insurance industry. We attribute this to increased employee morale as a result of the emphasis on employee welfare and wellness.
>
> Our wellness program is very broad and includes career training. We think the fact that we have a wellness program that includes a fitness center is an enormous recruiting tool. I think a company can have a very good program without putting in a gym. However, having the facilities sends out a strong message that there is an environmental aura that encourages everybody to take care of themselves. It says we care about weight management and stress reduction programs, that there is clear air here, and the food in the cafeteria is healthful and employees may choose to exercise.

With respect to results, one measure we have noted is cheerfulness and the look of health. Our informal studies show that our people who participate in wellness programs go to the doctor less frequently and are healthier. We know that people who smoke stay longer in the hospital. Studies show that for every dollar spent on fitness/wellness programs, companies are getting back two to six dollars in health care cost savings, reduced absenteeism, etc. Over half of disease and untimely deaths are caused by bad health habits. The most effective place to help people change habits is the workplace.

Electronic Data Systems

Electronic Data Systems notes that between 1984 and 1988 their LifeKey® program documented decreases in the number of employees who smoke and in absenteeism, while increases were observed for such variables as seat belt usage and healthier eating patterns. (For a further discussion of Electronic Data Systems' program, see Section II.)

General Motors

General Motors screened and rescreened some 325,000 employees for hypertension through 1987. Results showed that 18 percent of the employees had hypertension and one third of these were unaware of their condition. The potential savings in medical costs and absenteeism (in addition to the savings in lives and suffering) resulting from the detection of nearly 20,000 previously undetected cases of hypertension is staggering. (See Section II for a description of General Motors' corporate-wide health promotion program.)

Tenneco

William J. Bernacki, M.D., Vice President, Health, Environmental Medicine and Safety, Tenneco, Inc.,[13] spoke with us about the value versus the cost of fitness programs.

Our studies have shown that fitness programs are an excellent recruiting tool. We are a high technology company. Fitness is important to people working in such industries. If you want the high-level upbeat person, then you will have to offer these types of programs. Without these programs you will lose the best employees to your competitors.

The cost of a fitness program is very low. It should be looked upon as a benefit to recruit and retain bright people and this is justification enough. Our experience has been that almost all of the young, bright college grads sign up for our fitness programs.

Because we have such a large number of people exercising there is a sense of binding among employees. These are not just the body builders. It pulls together our entire company. Our program costs about $400,000 a year to run as opposed to the company aircraft which costs $17,000,000 +. It is very inexpensive and yields substantial results.

Like other companies, Tenneco is also interested in minimizing lower back problems. To achieve this goal they have initiated a creative "Hard Hats and Back" program, which is a healthy back program designed for the off-shore oil rig environment.

This body of data, although not intended to be statistically and methodologically rigorous, drives home a point made very well by Robert Rosen in his book, *Healthy Companies*,[14] namely, that a healthy organizational climate is a prerequisite to the successful implementation of health promotion programs. By "climate," we mean a corporate attitude toward the well-being of employees—something that cannot be measured statistically but is readily recognized by those companies that put people first.

The larger issue centers squarely on what Kenneth Warner calls the "uses and abuses of the economic argument." Warner[15] observes that

Health promotion programming is an excellent example of a function that addresses multiple business objectives, including better employee relations and stronger corporate image, as well as the economic well-being of the enterprise. A complete economic analysis must recognize all these elements.

At this point, Warner[16] maintains, the traditional view of health promotion has been focused on a "cost-containment mentality." The raison-d'etre of health promotion, however, is a quality of life for employees. From this perspective, which is humanistic, not strictly capitalistic, the future justifications of health promotion will focus more on the cost-effectiveness of programs than on the containment of costs.

WHAT'S AHEAD?

In order to appreciate the value of fitness/wellness programs as well as to assess the relative effectiveness of the systems used to deliver these programs, it is necessary to have a basic understanding of what it means to be fit and healthy. In addition, managers should be aware of the primary factors that contribute to good physical and mental well-being.

We provide this information in two ways. First, Chapter 3 explains the basics of "fitness"—what it is and is not—as well as some basics of exercise. The chapter also addresses the definition of being "healthy." A health style self-test is included, in addition to a copy of Hershey Foods' detailed medical history form, which may be used as a standard. Finally, Chapter 3 provides important information every manager should have concerning smoking and the control of blood pressure, weight, and cholesterol.

Section III, provided by William S. Frankl, M.D., provides detailed information for those managers who want to learn more about appropriate aerobic exercise, the types and recommended frequency of exercise, optimum heart rate, warming up, pre-exercise physical examinations, the effects of smoking, high blood pressure, cholesterol, weight, and alcohol on one's overall health, plus other topics that directly impact employee fitness and wellness. We strongly recommend studying this material from both a managerial and a personal perspective.

Second, Chapter 4 looks at the important health issue of stress from the manager's perspective. Stress has been linked with numerous health problems and is costing companies millions of dollars each year in lost productivity, absenteeism, medical expenses, and workers' compensation claims. Managers need to understand their effect on employees' stress levels and how management's interactions with employees play an integral part in employee fitness and health.

ENDNOTES

1. Kenneth E. Warner, Ph.D., "Selling Health Promotion to Corporate America: Uses and Abuses of the Economic Argument," *Health Education Quarterly,* 14(1987), p. 41.
2. U.S. Office of Technology Assessment, "Technology and the American Economic Transition: Choices for the Future—a Summary" (Washington, D.C.: U.S. Superintendent of Documents, 1988), p. 42.
3. Jerry M. Linenger, M.D., and Doris A. Abood, Ed.D., "Fighting Fit: An Organizational Behavior-Based Worksite Intervention Program," unpublished manuscript, 1987.
4. Ibid.
5. The American Heart Association, Greater Boston Division, *The Corporate Heart: Guidelines to Cardiovascular Health Promotion Programs in Business and Industry* (Boston: American Heart Assn., 1988), pp. 3–5.
6. Ibid.
7. American Diabetes Association, *"Working on Winning." A Wellness Program* (Alexandria, VA: American Diabetes Assn., Inc., 1988).
8. David R. Anderson, Ph.D., and William S. Jose II, Ph.D., "Employee Lifestyle and the Bottom Line: Results of the StayWell Evaluation," *Fitness in Business,* 3(1987), p. 86.
9. Victoria George and William E. Hembree, *Breakthroughs in Health-Care Management: Employer and Union Initiatives* (Elmsford, N.Y.: Pergamon Press, 1986), p. 34.
10. Ibid.
11. Statement provided to the authors by Fitness Systems.
12. Interview with William M. Kizer.
13. Interview with Edward J. Bernacki, M.D.
14. Robert H. Rosen, *Healthy Companies: A Human Resources Approach* (New York: American Management Associations, 1986).
15. Kenneth E. Warner, Ph.D., "Selling Health Promotion to Corporate America: Uses and Abuses of the Economic Argument," *Health Education Quarterly,* 14(1987), p. 41.
16. Ibid.

CHAPTER 3

WHAT MANAGERS NEED TO KNOW ABOUT FITNESS AND HEALTH

This is the law . . . that the strong shall
thrive, that surely the weak will
perish, and only the fit survive.
Robert W. Service

This chapter provides managers with the basic information they need to understand the concepts of fitness and good health within the context of the fitness/wellness movement. This chapter specifically examines the physical aspects of fitness and wellness, and Chapter 4 explains the various aspects of stress and stress management.

We note that, although the fitness/wellness movement is concerned primarily with exercise, weight management, alcohol control, personal safety, and other health issues, many executives and managers we interviewed take a much broader view of fitness and wellness. Especially among senior-level executives, the more traditional aspects of exercise, good nutrition, and control of alcohol and other substances are viewed as but one part of a larger definition of fitness and wellness that includes the ability to communicate, the knowledge to perform the job, and a positive self-image and spirit.

The executives described the need not only to help employees keep themselves physically fit and healthy, but also to help them keep up-to-date on the technical, communications, and interpersonal skills required to perform their jobs. Finally, these managers spoke to the need for providing a positive managerial attitude and work conditions which will enhance employee spirit.

These managers indicated the need for "spirited employees" and viewed employees in a broad context of physical, mental, and spiritual fitness. They spoke to us about the need for teamwork within organizations and the need for some rather profound changes in managerial attitudes.

Leo Beebe, Chairman and CEO of K-Tron International,[1] stated it this way:

> First, it is necessary to address the question of what is fitness. *Fitness includes body, brains and soul; it also includes the person's instincts, social conscience and ethics.* Anybody who thinks that fitness just refers to physical fitness is taking a very narrow viewpoint. It is necessary to develop people in three dimensions: body, mind and spirit.
>
> Fitness programs should not be implemented just for the sake of physical fitness. From my perspective, fitness programs should be a part of a total human engineering package designed to help people learn and grow throughout their careers.
>
> I think that to emphasize any of these things out of context is a mistake. I think it is foolish to run a fitness program just to have a fitness program that is something that is attractive and maybe a part of a little paternalistic effort.
>
> The fitness program should be woven into the fabric of the total human engineering approach. Furthermore, I don't think you can fool employees by saying we will back your softball team or give you a nice little exercise room and then cut them on some other things. The approach has to be comprehensive.

Based on our research and interviews, we envision a much more global view of total employee fitness in the future, with fitness/wellness programs as we know them today being closely integrated with various corporate training programs.

THE MEANING OF PHYSICAL FITNESS AND GOOD HEALTH

> The health of nations is more
> important than the wealth of
> nations.
> *Will Durant*

What does it mean to be physically fit and in good health? This is a very difficult question to answer; responses vary from person to person. Consider physical fitness first. Based on our studies and Dr. Frankl's suggestions in Section III, we conclude that being physically "fit" for most people means being able to undertake aerobic exercise three or four times per week for a half hour at a heart rate that is 60 to 75 percent of 220 less the person's age, which is the American Heart Association's target heart rate. (For a discussion of aerobic exercise, see Section III.) In all cases, the actual target rate should be established by a physician and based upon individual assessment, taking into account the individual's age and the possibility of underlying heart disease.

Based on our interviews, this definition of a physically "fit" person seems to be a reasonable baseline for most people. Others would disagree, however. The "Adult Fitness Standards" provided by the President's Council on Physical Fitness & Sports, for example, recommends various anaerobic, as well as aerobic, exercises.

It is important to note that being physically fit with respect to exercising regularly does not mean that a person necessarily is "fit" to install a new roof on the house, replace the front sidewalk, or shovel snow. These kinds of physical activities are anaerobic in nature and not only place great stress on the cardiovascular system, but also can cause back or other injuries. Being "fit," therefore, should not suggest taking on projects that involve anaerobic exercise. Take note, too, that the "fit" person who regularly rides a bike, for example, should not do so in very hot or cold weather.

Is the baseline exercise program right for everyone? The answer is no. Some people may have physical conditions that limit their ability to exercise. Accordingly, they may have to start with a very low level of exercise and work toward achieving the baseline rate. Others may have specific needs for particular muscular strength or flexibility. For example, a person who lifts heavy objects should follow a regular program of warm-up and muscle stretching prior to lifting. Such a properly directed program has the potential of greatly reducing back injuries.

Some people whose work is physical in nature believe that they do not need to participate in regular aerobic exercises. In fact, most physical work is anaerobic in nature. It places the heart and other muscles under high levels of stress for short periods of time. Consequently, even though a person has a job involving physical activity, that person likely still needs regular aerobic exercise. This should be discussed with a physician.

Are bulging muscles a sign of physical fitness? The experts don't think so. "Toning up" certain muscle groups is an important component in overall physical fitness, but developing a "muscle magazine" physique is hardly synonymous with physical fitness. Indeed, caution is indicated in the use of isometric or anaerobic exercises, since these can be very stressful to the cardiovascular system. In general, regular aerobic exercise is best for nearly everyone and will produce good muscle tone.

Finally, *everyone should have an appropriate physical examination before starting an exercise program.* Also, it is important to always warm up before exercising and cool down after exercising and spread the exercise periods out over the week. The exercise program preferably should be under the direction of an exercise physiologist or a physician. Also, the choice of an aerobic exercise should be based on an activity that is enjoyable, preferably one that can be easily integrated into a person's normal lifestyle.

What constitutes being healthy? The experts we interviewed say that being healthy is literally feeling healthy—possessing a positive state of mind about one's body that comes from a sensible, balanced program aimed at appropriate levels of exercise, proper diet, and blood pressure control, as well as avoidance of activities and substances that abuse the body.

How does one get to feel healthy? One way is to exercise regularly as described above and not to abuse the body. What else should a person do to keep healthy? The experts we interviewed suggest the following:

1. Don't smoke.
2. Maintain weight within reasonable limits.
3. Maintain cholesterol under 200, as appropriate.
4. Limit or eliminate alcohol consumption.
5. Eat well-balanced meals.
6. Learn to deal with stress (not all stress is "bad").
7. Have physical exams at appropriate intervals.
8. Do not use any nonprescription drugs and follow doctor's instructions when using prescription drugs.
9. Enjoy life, take things less seriously, and laugh more often!

We will discuss some of these in more detail later in the chapter.

ASSESSING PHYSICAL FITNESS AND WELLNESS

*In life as in a football game, the
principle to follow is: Hit the
hard line.*
Theodore Roosevelt

We begin this section with a self-assessment test that can be used by employees to assess their physical fitness and wellness. Based on the result of this test, employees are encouraged to select the components of their lifestyles that they need to change in order to improve their physical fitness and make and keep them "well."

After reviewing the self-assessment test, refer to the "Medical History Preventive Medical Program" questionnaire provided by Hershey Foods Corporation, which is included at the end of this chapter. Most employees can answer many of the questions included in the "Medical History." If you use a questionnaire such as this one, it is important to encourage employees to have their doctors review their answers. A good time to do this is at their next physical examination. The combined results of the self-assessment test and Hershey Foods' "Medical History" will provide an extremely comprehensive baseline for starting or enhancing your company's personal physical fitness and wellness program.

HEALTH STYLE: A SELF-TEST

The following self-test, which was developed by the U.S. Health Department, is not "pass-fail." It is simply an indicator of how well a person is doing in his or her quest to stay healthy. The test has six sections: smoking, alcohol and drugs, nutrition, exercise and fitness, stress control, and safety. The person taking the test completes one section at a time by circling the number corresponding to the answer that best describes his or her behavior (2 for "Almost Always," 1 for "Sometimes," and 0 for "Almost Never"). Then the person adds the numbers circled and writes the score on the line provided at the end of each section. The highest score for each section is 10.

A Test for Better Health

	Almost Always	Sometimes	Almost Never
I. Cigarette Smoking			
If you never smoke, enter a score of 10 for this section and go to the next section on Alcohol and Drugs.			
1. I avoid smoking cigarettes.	2	1	0
2. I smoke only low tar and nicotine cigarettes or I smoke a pipe or cigars.	2	1	0
Smoking Score _____			
II. Alcohol and Drugs			
1. I avoid drinking alcoholic beverages or I drink no more than 1 or 2 drinks a day.	4	1	0
2. I avoid using alcohol or other drugs (especially illegal drugs) as a way of handling stressful situations or the problems of my life.	2	1	0
3. I am careful not to drink alcohol when taking certain medicines or when pregnant.	2	1	0
4. I read and follow the label directions when using prescribed and over-the-counter drugs.	2	1	0
Alcohol and Drug Score _____			
III. Eating Habits			
1. I eat a variety of foods each day, such as fruits and vegetables, whole grain breads and cereals, lean meats, dairy products, dry peas and beans, and nuts and peas.	4	1	0
2. I limit the amount of fat, saturated fat, and cholesterol I eat.	2	1	0

A Test for Better Health (*continued*)

	Almost Always	Sometimes	Almost Never
3. I limit the amount of salt I eat by cooking with only small amounts, not adding salt at the table, and avoiding salty snacks.	2	1	0
4. I avoid eating too much sugar (especially frequent snacks of sticky candy or soft drinks).	2	1	0

Eating Habits Score _____

IV. Exercise/Fitness

	Almost Always	Sometimes	Almost Never
1. I maintain a desired weight, avoiding overweight and underweight.	3	1	0
2. I do vigorous exercises for 15–30 minutes at least 3 times a week (running, swimming, brisk walking).	3	1	0
3. I do exercises that enhance my muscle tone for 15–30 minutes at least 3 times a week (calisthenics, yoga).	2	1	0
4. I use part of my leisure time participating in individual, family, or team activities that increase my level of fitness (gardening, bowling, golf, baseball).	2	1	0

Execise/Fitness Score _____

V. Stress Control

	Almost Always	Sometimes	Almost Never
1. I have a job or do other work that I enjoy.	2	1	0
2. I find it easy to relax and express my feelings.	2	1	0
3. I recognize early, and prepare for, events or situation likely to be stressful to me.	2	1	0
4. I have close friends, relatives, or others whom I can talk to about personal matters and call on for help.	2	1	0
5. I participate in group activities (such as church and community organizations) or hobbies that I enjoy.	2	1	0

Stress Control Score _____

A Test for Better Health (*concluded*)

	Almost Always	Sometimes	Almost Never
VI. Safety			
1. I wear a seat belt while riding in a car.	2	1	0
2. I avoid driving while under the influence of alcohol and other drugs.	2	1	0
3. I obey traffic rules and the speed limit.	2	1	0
4. I am careful when using potentially harmful products or substances (cleaners, poisons).	2	1	0
5. I avoid smoking in bed.	2	1	0
			Safety Score _____

Remember, there is no total score for this test. You should look at each section separately to identify aspects of your lifestyle that may need improvement or change.

What the Scores Mean

Scores of 9 and 10: Excellent! You are putting your knowledge to work for you by practicing good health habits. As long as you continue to do so, this area should not pose a serious health risk.

Scores of 6 to 8: Your health habits are good, but a need for some improvement is indicated. What changes could you make to improve your score? Even small changes are worth considering!

Scores of 3 to 5: You're in the danger zone. You should seriously think about changing your lifestyle.

Scores 0 to 2: You clearly are taking serious and unnecessary health risks. Immediate intervention is warranted.

FIGURE 3–1
Your Healthstyle Scores

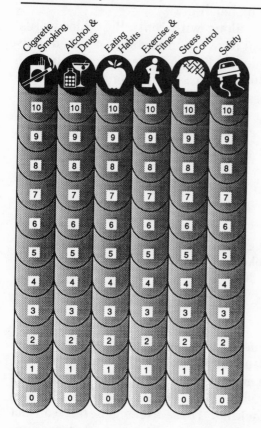

BASIC HEALTH FACTORS

> He who has health, has hope; and he who
> has hope has everything.

In this and the following sections of this chapter, we briefly discuss four key health factors in all fitness/wellness programs: not smoking, blood pressure control, weight control, and blood cholesterol level control. Most people can manage these four critical health factors through a combination of self-discipline, diet and exercise. By controlling them a person can increase the capacity for exercise, add to longevity, improve appearance, and enhance the quality of his or her life.

Although not smoking, along with controlling blood pressure, weight, and cholesterol are very important for all employees, it is essential that employees be able to deal effectively with stress—both in the workplace and in their personal lives. In the following chapter we discuss stress from a management perspective and provide a detailed stress questionnaire that employees can use to identify those areas, such as job, life, and family, which produce and reduce stress.

NOT SMOKING

> It's hard to say who brags
> more, the reformed smoker or
> the guy whose car gets 30
> miles to the gallon.
> *James Alexander Thom*

Smoking is the number-one risk factor in coronary artery disease and is very offensive to many people. Furthermore, passive smoking (just being in a room where other people smoke) is almost as hazardous as smoking. Consequently, most companies have limited areas for smoking. These areas generally do not include meeting rooms and open office areas and often are limited to hallways and similar areas. Programs aimed at reducing the level of employee smoking should be a first priority in fitness/wellness programs.

HIGH BLOOD PRESSURE

> When the cup is full, carry
> it even.

Companies regularly check for high blood pressure (hypertension) when they give preemployment physical exams. This is an excellent idea because many people have no idea that they have hypertension. High blood pressure is literally the silent killer.

It is important that all employees know their blood pressure and take steps to keep it under control. Although high blood pressure increases the risk of heart attack and stroke, it can be controlled in most people. The American Heart Association reports that *"15% to 20% of adults have abnormally elevated blood pressure. (Greater than 140/90 mm/Hg.)."* High blood pressure affects vital body areas, particularly the heart, brain, and kidneys. In addition to making the heart pump harder, high blood pressure also lessens the elasticity of arteries, which can lead to a heart attack. High blood pressure also speeds up the process of atherosclerosis (hardening of the arteries) and, by increasing wear on the retina's blood vessels, can damage the eyes. Finally, high blood pressure results in strokes for many people. For these reasons, all employees need to keep their blood pressure under control.

Factors Contributing to High Blood Pressure

Several factors contribute to high blood pressure. Managers should be aware of these factors so that they can avoid high blood pressure and help employees to do likewise. The primary factors are listed below:

1. Heredity
Unfortunately, a person's resume is already written in this area! If a parent or a sibling has high blood pressure, it is especially important to have blood pressure monitored regularly. Note also that blacks are more affected than whites—one in four blacks has the disease, which makes it the biggest single cause of death within this group.

2. Emotions
When a person is angry or fearful, his or her blood pressure goes up—that's natural. Some people, however, get accustomed to responding to events in daily life as if they were all emergencies. This has the effect of keeping their blood pressure abnormally high much of the time. Learning how to effectively deal with stress, as well as learning what causes stress, can have a positive effect on controlling blood pressure.

3. Smoking
Heavy cigarette smoking is implicated in high blood pressure. Nicotine is known to raise blood pressure. Smoking, of course, has also been directly related to increased incidence of heart disease and is now strongly discouraged by many companies. If your company has a smoking cessation plan, encourage employees to take advantage of it and stop smoking now.

4. Diet
High salt diets certainly contribute to hypertension. Following Dr. Frankl's advice in the Medical Component at the end of this book, along with avoiding putting salt on foods and using less salt when cooking, will help to reduce high blood pressure.

High levels of cholesterol may lead to acceleration of atherosclerosis and therefore to higher blood pressure. Accordingly, controlling cholesterol is important to reducing blood pressure or keeping blood pressure from increasing.

5. Weight
Overweight people tend to have high blood pressure.

6. Exercise
People who do not exercise regularly tend to have higher blood pressure than those who do. People who do exercise usually weigh less and have better control over their reactions to stress. Appropriate exercise is crucial to good health.

High blood pressure is most prelavent among men and usually appears for the first time between ages 35 and 55. Women who have never had high blood pressure may develop it during pregnancy. For some women, the use of certain contraceptives increases the level of estrogen and thereby causes high blood pressure.

Blood Pressure Screening

Since many people with high blood pressure are completely unaware of it, it is very important that all employees be screened regularly. Many of the companies we surveyed already provide regular blood pressure screening.

Controlling High Blood Pressure

If a person has high blood pressure, he or she may be able to control it by increasing exercise, losing weight, moderating alcohol consumption, decreasing salt intake, avoiding tobacco, and/or consuming less dietary saturated fat. Treatment should be under the direction of a physician, who in some cases may prescribe medication.

WEIGHT MANAGEMENT

> To succeed, keep on doing what it
> took to get started.

Being overweight can have a real impact on a person's health. Being overweight is associated with high blood pressure, increased levels of blood fats (triglycerides) and cholesterol, heart disease, strokes, the most common type of diabetes, and certain cancers.

Since there is prejudice against fat people (both off and on the job), the overweight employee can suffer from added stress. Also, since being overweight is associated with other health risk factors, you should encourage overweight employees to participate in medically supervised weight reduction programs.

You should be aware that *many diet books offer advice that is medically unsound, may be harmful to one's health, and will likely provide only temporary results. If a person has a weight problem, the solution is changing eating habits, preferably while starting or expanding an exercise program.* Some practical suggestions for weight reduction are discussed below.

Exercise and Weight Management—The Interaction

First, it is important to understand the relationship between exercise and weight control. Exercise is very important to weight reduction for five reasons:

1. *Exercising actually reduces appetite for many people,* and so a person may not feel as hungry if he or she exercises.

2. *Exercising burns calories,* which means less dieting to achieve the same weight-reduction goals.

3. *Exercising tends to produce a natural emotional high.* Since many people eat excessively when they are upset or depressed, exercising can reduce the need for those excess calories.

4. *Exercising provides an energy boost.* Many people snack to increase their energy. Exercise is more effective than eating and burns calories rather than adding them.

5. *Exercising tones the skin and muscles,* which is important when losing weight. Without concurrent exercise, skin may tend to hang loosely and detract from the dieter's appearance.

Weight Loss Programs

The equation for losing weight is very simple: a person must take in fewer calories than he or she burns. This usually means decreasing food consumption or changing eating patterns while increasing physical activity. There are three basic steps in the control of overeating:

- Eat slowly.
- Take smaller portions.
- Avoid "seconds."

For most people who decide to lose weight, a steady loss of one to two pounds a week—until he or she reaches the desired weight—is safe. At the beginning of a weight-reduction diet, much of the weight loss comes from loss of water. Long-term success depends on new and better habits of eating and exercise. That is why so-called *fad* and *crash diets* usually fail in the long run. In addition, they may endanger the dieter's health.

Employees should be discouraged from losing weight too quickly. They should avoid crash diets that severely restrict the variety of foods allowed. Diets containing fewer than 800 calories per day may be hazardous and should be undertaken only under medical supervision. Many people who follow such diets for several days many find themselves "pigging out" and eating more in the long run than they would have if they had followed a sensible diet and exercise program.

Also, attempting to lose weight by inducing vomiting or by taking laxatives is very dangerous. Vomiting and purging can cause a chemical imbalance that can lead to irregular heartbeat and even death.

The following general guidelines are most productive in weight loss programs:

- Eat a variety of foods that are low in calories and high in nutrients.
- Eat more fruits.
- Eat less fat and fatty foods.
- Increase the intake of complex carbohydrates, as opposed to refined, processed carbohydrates.
- Drink fewer alcoholic beverages (or eliminate alcohol entirely).
- Increase physical activity.

Most people who report successful weight loss programs have changed their diet and exercise patterns gradually. *Quick changes in either eating or exercise habits may be unhealthy, and the dieter likely will revert to old patterns because the changes will produce unpleasant stresses in his or her life. Long-term lifestyle changes seldom come rapidly.* The experts we interviewed indicate that behavior modification usually takes a minimum of three weeks—frequently more. So, one should not expect immediate results when trying to lose weight. Quick changes are neither healthy nor are they likely to be long-lasting.

CHOLESTEROL

Success is a ladder which cannot
be climbed with your hands in your
pockets.

Cholesterol is another key factor in an employee's total fitness profile that can be controlled. As Dr. Frankl notes, a cholesterol level of 200 or less generally is desirable.

Men generally have higher cholesterol counts than women.

Women tend to have higher high-density lipoproteins (HDL), or "good" cholesterol counts, which may account for the fact that a women's chance of developing heart disease is about one third that of a man.

Diet and Cholesterol

In many instances it is possible to reduce one's low-density lipoproteins (LDL), or "bad" cholesterol level by changing diet and to increase the HDL level by exercising. Experts recommend limiting cholesterol intake to 300 milligrams per day. An egg, for example, has 270 milligrams. Since cholesterol is found only in foods from animals (including egg yolks, meat, fish, poultry, and whole mile products), avoiding these, along with commercial baked goods made with lard (such as doughnuts, cookies, and cake) and processed lunch meats, will help to reduce the amount of serum cholesterol. Also, saturated fats (those which are normally hard at room temperature) should be avoided. Many processed foods undergo a process called "hydrogenation," which produces saturated fats. Processed foods therefore should be avoided as well.

Fruits, vegetables, starches, and grain cereals contain no cholesterol and little saturated fats. Vegetable oils are free of cholesterol, and most contain large amounts of polyunsaturated fats. Polyunsaturated fats and monounsaturated fats (such as corn and safflower oil) tend to reduce blood cholesterol levels.

Changing dietary patterns can be a difficult task. Our research indicates that radical changes in eating habits may be both unhealthy and short lasting. As noted above, modifications, rather than changes, should be considered. In discussing weight reduction programs with employees, you might suggest, for example, changing gradually from whole milk to low-fat and finally to nonfat milk. Instead of eating fast-food burgers and fries, employees should be encouraged to try the salad bar, or make a tuna sandwich and have an apple for desert. Switching from eggs with ham and sausage at breakfast to a whole grain cereal with fruit and skim milk is another good choice. Of course, as a manager, you can provide a "healthy" eating example for others as well as encourage employees to participate in company-sponsored weight control programs.

WHAT'S AHEAD?

In Chapter 4, we examine stress from the perspective of company leadership. We discuss the costs of stress, how managers view personal and on-the-job stress, and what managers do to deal with stress. Our findings have broad implications for managers and employees alike and provide a foundation for a new look at how managers and subordinates interact and communicate.

APPENDIX A

MEDICAL HISTORY
PREVENTIVE MEDICAL PROGRAM
HERSHEY FOODS CORPORATION

Appendix A, pages 50–62, contains the medical history forms used by the employees of the Hershey Foods Corporation.

CONFIDENTIAL

MEDICAL HISTORY
PREVENTIVE MEDICAL PROGRAM

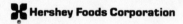 **Hershey Foods Corporation**

THE OBJECTIVES OF THIS EXAMINATION ARE TO EVALUATE THE PRESENT STATE OF YOUR HEALTH AND DETECT THE PRESENCE OF ANY DISORDER OR CONDITION WHICH COULD LEAD TO ILLNESS IN THE FUTURE. IT IS NOT INTENDED TO REPLACE EXAMINATIONS BY YOUR PERSONAL PHYSICIAN AND SHOULD NOT INTERRUPT ANY REGULAR PATTERN OF CARE OR TREATMENT BY YOUR DOCTOR. PLEASE ANSWER THE QUESTIONS AS OBJECTIVELY AND FRANKLY AS YOU CAN, BECAUSE A COMPLETE AND ACCURATE MEDICAL HISTORY IS ESSENTIAL. YOUR COMPLETED QUESTIONAIRE WILL ENABLE THE EXAMINING PHYSICIAN TO CONCENTRATE ON THOSE ASPECTS OF YOUR HEALTH WHICH ARE MOST IMPORTANT. IF YOUR ARE UNCERTAIN ABOUT HOW YOU SHOULD ANSWER ANY QUESTION, LEAVE IT UNANSWERED.

PLEASE RETURN IT AT THE TIME OF YOUR APPOINTMENT. ALL OF THE INFORMATION WILL BE KEPT STRICTLY **CONFIDENTIAL** AND WILL **NOT** BE **REVEALED** TO ANYONE **WITHOUT YOUR CONSENT**. A REPORT OF THE RESULTS WILL BE SENT TO YOUR HOME.

NAME	DATE

HOME ADDRESS	PHONE: HOME- WORK-

CITY	STATE	ZIP CODE	COUNTRY

DATE OF BIRTH	MALE ☐ FEMALE ☐	SINGLE ☐ MARRIED ☐	DIVORCED ☐ SEPARATED ☐

OCCUPATION/JOB TITLE	YEARS EMPLOYED BY HFC

NAME OF YOUR PERSONAL PHYSICIAN

ADDRESS

CITY	STATE	ZIP CODE

DO YOU WANT A COPY OF THE REPORT OF THIS EXAMINATION SENT TO YOUR DOCTOR? YES ☐ NO ☐

(REV 7/87)

1. DO YOU HAVE ANY PHYSICAL COMPLAINTS OR DISABILITIES AT THE PRESENT? IF SO, PLEASE DESCRIBE THEM:

_____

_____

_____

_____

_____

2. ARE YOU TAKING ANY MEDICINE , DRUGS (PILLS), INJECTIONS, ETC. IF SO, PLEASE LIST THEM WITH THE DOSAGE.

MEDICINE	DOSE	HOW OFTEN TAKEN

3. HAVE YOU CONSULTED OR BEEN TREATED BY CLINCS, PHYSICIANS, OR OTHER PRACTITIONERS WITHIN THE PAST 5 YEARS? IF SO, LIST THEM:

YEAR	DOCTOR	TREATED FOR

4. IF YOU WERE EVER HOSPITALIZED OR OPERATED UPON, PLEASE LIST BELOW:

YEAR	DIAGNOSIS OR CAUSE FOR HOSPITALIZATION	SURGICAL OPERATIONS

5. DO YOU HAVE/HAVE YOU HAD:
   - -HEART DISEASE? YES☐ NO☐
   - -A HEART MURMUR? YES☐ NO☐
       - FROM BIRTH- YES☐ NO☐   DURING PREGNANCY- YES☐ NO☐
       - LIMITING-ACTIVITY YES☐ NO☐   NEEDING TREATMENT- YES☐ NO☐
   - -AN ENLARGED HEART? YES☐ NO☐
   - -A HEART ATTACK (CORONARY, INFARCT)?   YES☐ NO☐ IF SO, GIVE DATE(S):
   - -AN ABNORMAL ELECTROCARDIOGRAM (ECG, EKG)? YES☐ NO☐ IF SO, GIVE DATE:
   - -HEART SURGERY? YES☐ NO☐ IF SO, TYPE: DATE:

6. DO YOU HAVE SHORTNESS OF BREATH: YES☐ NO☐
   - WITH YOUR USUAL WORK OR ACTIVITY? YES☐ NO☐
   - THAT MAKES YOU STOP AFTER CLIMBING 10-14 STEPS? YES☐ NO☐

7. DO YOU HAVE REPEATED PAIN OR PRESSURE OR TIGHT FEELING IN YOUR CHEST? YES☐ NO☐
   - ASSOCIATED WITH EXERCISE? YES☐ NO☐   THAT AWAKENS YOU FROM SLEEP? YES☐ NO☐
   - ASSOCIATED WITH ANGER? YES☐ NO☐   WHEN YOU WALK UPHILL? YES☐ NO☐

8. IN THE PAST SIX MONTHS HAVE YOU HAD:
   - THUMPING, RACING OR IRREGULARITY OF THE HEART? YES☐ NO☐
   - AWAKENING AT NIGHT DUE TO SHORTNESS OF BREATH? YES☐ NO☐
   - PAINLESS SWELLING OF BOTH FEET OR BOTH ANKLES? YES☐ NO☐

(✔) YES NO

9. HAVE YOU GAINED OR LOST 5 POUNDS OR MORE WITHIN THE PAST 6 MONTHS? ☐ ☐
10. HAVE YOU HAD CHILLS OR FEVER RECENTLY? ☐ ☐
11. HAVE YOU NOTICED ANY SWELLING OR LUMP IN YOUR NECK, ARMPITS, GROIN OR ELSEWHERE? ☐ ☐
12. HAVE YOU EVER WORN GLASSES, OR BEEN ADVISED TO WEAR THEM? ☐ ☐
13. ARE YOU HAVING INCREASING DIFFICULTY READING SMALL PRINT, OR SEEING THINGS AT A DISTANCE? ☐ ☐
14. HAVE YOU HAD ANY BLURRING, HAZINESS, OR CLOUDING OF YOUR VISION OR DO YOU SEE "HALOS" AROUND LIGHTS? ☐ ☐
15. DO YOU HAVE ANY BLIND SPOTS IN YOUR VISION? ☐ ☐
16. DO YOU HAVE DIFFICULTY SEEING OUT OF THE "CORNER OF YOUR EYE" AS WELL AS YOU USED TO? ☐ ☐
17. HAVE YOU EVER HAD BLINDNESS OR PARTIAL BLINDNESS? ☐ ☐
18. HAVE YOU HAD ANY PAIN OR INFLAMMATION IN YOUR EYES WITHIN THE PAST YEAR? ☐ ☐
19. DO YOU OCCASIONALLY SEE A SPOT OR SPOTS IN FRONT OF YOUR EYES? ☐ ☐
20. DID YOU EVER SEE DOUBLE? ☐ ☐
21. HAVE YOU EVER SUSPECTED OR BEEN TOLD YOU WERE COLOR BLIND? ☐ ☐
22. HAVE YOU HAD ANY LOSS OF HEARING? ☐ ☐
23. HAVE YOU HAD EARACHES OR DISCHARGE FROM YOUR EARS IN RECENT YEARS? ☐ ☐

(✔) YES NO

24. DO YOU HAVE BUZZING OR RINGING IN YOUR EARS? ☐ ☐
25. DO YOU BECOME SICK EASILY FROM THE MOTION OF A CAR, TRAIN, PLANE, OR SHIP? ☐ ☐
26. DO YOU HAVE MORE THAN TWO OR THREE "COLDS" PER YEAR? ☐ ☐
27. DO YOU HAVE CHRONIC DISCHARGE FROM YOUR NOSE? ☐ ☐
28. DO YOU HAVE FREQUENT OR SEVERE NOSEBLEEDS? ☐ ☐
29. DO YOU HAVE DIFFICULTY BREATHING THROUGH EITHER SIDE OF YOUR NOSE? ☐ ☐
30. HAVE YOU EVER HAD SINUS TROUBLE? ☐ ☐
31. DO YOU HAVE DIFFICULTY RECOGNIZING COMMON ODORS AS WELL AS YOU USED TO? ☐ ☐
32. DO YOU HAVE FREQUENT OR SEVERE SORE THROAT? ☐ ☐
33. DO YOU HAVE TO CLEAR YOUR THROAT OFTEN? ☐ ☐
34. HAS IT BEEN MORE THAN A YEAR SINCE YOU WERE EXAMINED BY A DENTIST? ☐ ☐
35. HAVE YOU BEEN HOARSE RECENTLY OR HAD TROUBLE SWALLOWING? ☐ ☐
36. DO YOU HAVE A CHRONIC COUGH? ☐ ☐
37. DO YOU COUGH UP PHLEGM? ☐ ☐
38. HAVE YOU EVER COUGHED UP BLOOD? ☐ ☐
39. DO YOU EVER NOTICE A WHEEZE IN YOUR CHEST ON BREATHING? ☐ ☐
40. HAVE YOU EVER BEEN TOLD YOU HAD LUNG OR BRONCHIAL TROUBLE? ☐ ☐
41. HAVE YOU EVER HAD CONTACT WITH A PERSON ILL WITH TUBERCULOSIS? ☐ ☐

	(✓) YES NO		(✓) YES NO
42. DO YOU HAVE NIGHT SWEATS?	☐ ☐	73. HAVE YOU EVER SUSPECTED OR BEEN TOLD YOU HAD A RUPTURE OR HERNIA?	☐ ☐
43. DO YOU GET PAIN IN YOUR NECK, SHOULDERS, OR ARMS?	☐ ☐	74. HAVE YOU BEEN TOLD YOU HAD KIDNEY OR BLADDER DISEASE?	☐ ☐
44. DO YOU FEET OR ANKLES SWELL?	☐ ☐	75. ARE YOU NOW HAVING TO PASS YOUR URINE MORE OFTEN THAN FORMERLY?	☐ ☐
45. HAVE YOU EVER BEEN TOLD YOU HAD HIGH BLOOD PRESSURE?	☐ ☐	76. DO YOU HAVE TO GET UP MOST NIGHTS TO URINATE? IF SO, HOW OFTEN? _____	☐ ☐
46. DO YOU HAVE VARICOSE VEINS?	☐ ☐	77. DO YOU HAVE ANY BURNING OR DISCOMFORT WHEN YOU URINATE?	☐ ☐
47. DO YOU EVER GET CRAMPS IN YOUR CALVES WHEN WALKING?	☐ ☐	78. DO YOU HAVE TROUBLE STARTING OR STOPPING YOUR URINE STREAM?	☐ ☐
48. DO YOUR HANDS EVER BECOME UNUSUALLY PALE, COLD, OR DISCOLORED?	☐ ☐	79. DO YOU EVER PASS URINE UNINTENTIONALLY?	☐ ☐
49. DO YOUR GUMS BLEED EASILY?	☐ ☐	80. HAVE YOUR EVER PASSED STONES OR GRAVEL IN YOUR URINE?	☐ ☐
50. IS YOUR TONGUE OFTEN SORE OR SENSITIVE?	☐ ☐	81. HAVE YOU EVER NOTICED OR BEEN TOLD THAT YOUR URINE CONTAINED BLOOD?	☐ ☐
51. HAVE YOU NOTICED ANY LOSS OF APPETITE?	☐ ☐	82. HAVE YOU EVER BEEN TOLD YOUR URINE CONTAINED PUS, ALBUMIN OR SUGAR?	☐ ☐
52. HAVE YOU HAD NAUSEA OR VOMITING RECENTLY?	☐ ☐	83. DO YOU HAVE TO PASS MUCH LARGER AMOUNTS OF URINE THAN FORMERLY?	☐ ☐
53. HAVE YOU EVER VOMITED BLOOD?	☐ ☐	84. HAVE YOU EVER HAD AN X-RAY EXAMINATION OF YOUR KIDNEYS OR URINARY BLADDER?	☐ ☐
54. DO YOU HAVE DIFFICULTY SWALLOWING?	☐ ☐	85. HAVE YOU EVER HAD A VENEREAL DISEASE?	☐ ☐
55. DO YOU HAVE EXCESSIVE GAS?	☐ ☐	86. DO YOUR FEET TROUBLE YOU IN ANY WAY?	☐ ☐
56. DO YOU HAVE ANY PAIN OR DISCOMFORT IN YOUR ABDOMEN?	☐ ☐	87. HAVE YOU HAD TROUBLE OF ANY SORT WITH YOUR BACK?	☐ ☐
57. HAVE YOU EVER BEEN TOLD YOU HAD AN ULCER?	☐ ☐	88. HAVE YOU EVER HAD AN X-RAY EXAMINATION OF YOUR BACK OR SPINE?	☐ ☐
58. HAVE YOU EVER BEEN TOLD YOU HAD GALLBLADDER TROUBLE OR GALLSTONES?	☐ ☐	89. HAVE YOU HAD ANY STIFFNESS, SWELLING, OR PAINS IN ANY OF YOUR JOINTS?	☐ ☐
59. ARE THERE ANY FOODS OR BEVERAGES WHICH UPSET YOU, OR WHICH YOU CANNOT TOLERATE?	☐ ☐	90. HAVE YOU EVER BEEN TOLD YOU HAD BURSITIS?	☐ ☐
60. ARE YOU ON A SPECIAL DIET OF ANY TYPE?	☐ ☐	91. DO YOU HAVE PERSISTENT HEADACHES?	☐ ☐
61. HAVE YOU EVER BEEN JAUNDICED (HAD YOUR SKIN OR THE WHITES OF YOUR EYES TURN YELLOW)?	☐ ☐	92. DO YOU HAVE FREQUENT OR SEVERE HEADACHES?	☐ ☐
62. HAVE YOU EVER HAD INTESTINAL WORMS OR PARASITES?	☐ ☐	93. HAVE YOU EVER BEEN TOLD YOU HAD NEURALGIA OR NEURITIS?	☐ ☐
63. ARE YOU OFTEN CONSTIPATED?	☐ ☐	94. HAVE YOU EVER HAD A PERSISTANT NUMBNESS OR WEAKNESS ANY PLACE IN YOUR BODY?	☐ ☐
64. HAVE YOU HAD DIARRHEA RECENTLY?	☐ ☐	95. WAS ANY PART OF YOUR BODY EVER PARALYZED?	☐ ☐
65. DO YOU HAVE LOOSE OR UNUSUALLY FREQUENT BOWEL MOVEMENTS?	☐ ☐	96. HAVE YOU EVER FAINTED?	☑ ☐
66. HAVE YOUR BOWEL HABITS CHANGED RECENTLY?	☐ ☐	97. HAVE YOU FELT LIGHT-HEADED OR DIZZY RECENTLY?	☐ ☐
67. HAVE YOU EVER PASSED BLOOD FROM YOUR RECTUM?	☐ ☐	98. HAVE YOU EVER HAD A SPELL, FIT OR CONVULSION? (EPILEPSY)	☐ ☐
68. DO YOUR BOWELS FUNCTION ANY DIFFERNTLY NOW THAN THEY DID 6 MONTHS OR A YEAR AGO?	☐ ☐	99. HAVE YOU EVER HAD A BRAIN-WAVE TRACING (ELECTROENCEPHALOGRAPHY)?	☐ ☐
69. ARE YOUR BOWEL MOVEMENTS EVER BLACK, WHITE, OR LIGHT GRAY IN COLOR?	☐ ☐	100. HAVE YOU EXPERIENCED ANY UNSTEADINESS IN YOUR WALKING OR BALANCE?	☐ ☐
70. HAVE YOU EVER PASSED MUCUS IN YOUR BOWEL MOVEMENTS?	☐ ☐		
71. HAVE YOU EVER HAD HEMORRHOIDS (PILES)?	☐ ☐		
72. HAVE YOU EVER HAD AN X-RAY EXAMINATION OF YOUR STOMACH, COLON OR GALLBLADDER?	☐ ☐		

(✓)
YES NO

101. HAVE YOU NOTICED ANY TREMOR, OR SHAKING OF YOUR HANDS OR ANY OTHER PART OF YOUR BODY? ☐ ☐

102. HAVE YOU EVER BEEN KNOCKED UNCONSCIOUS? ☐ ☐

103. HAS YOUR HANDWRITING CHANGED RECENTLY? ☐ ☐

104. DO YOU FIND IT MORE DIFFICULT TO CONCENTRATE THAN FORMERLY? ☐ ☐

105. IS IT DIFFICULT FOR YOU TO MAKE UP YOUR MIND? ☐ ☐

106. IS IT BECOMING MORE DIFFICULT FOR YOU TO REMEMBER THINGS? ☐ ☐

107. HAVE YOUR SLEEPING HABITS CHANGED RECENTLY? ☐ ☐

108. DO YOU OFTEN HAVE DIFFICULTY FALLING ASLEEP? ☐ ☐

109. DO YOU HAVE DIFFICULTY STAYING ASLEEP? ☐ ☐

110. DO YOU OFTEN FEEL TIRED AFTER AN AVERAGE NIGHT'S SLEEP? ☐ ☐

111. DO YOU TIRE VERY EASILY, OR OFTEN FEEL WEAK? ☐ ☐

112. DO YOU OFTEN HAVE DIFFICULTY REMAINING AWAKE DURING YOUR USUAL WAKING HOURS? ☐ ☐

113. ARE YOU SHY OR SENSITIVE? ☐ ☐

114. ARE YOUR FEELINGS HURT EASILY? ☐ ☐

115. ARE YOU OFTEN RESTLESS? ☐ ☐

116. ARE YOU "KEYED UP" MUCH OF THE TIME? ☐ ☐

117. IS IT DIFFICULT FOR YOU TO RELAX? ☐ ☐

118. ARE YOU EASILY IRRITATED AND UPSET? ☐ ☐

119. ARE YOU OFTEN DEPRESSED OR BLUE? ☐ ☐

120. DO YOU CRY EASILY? ☐ ☐

121. DO YOU HAVE ANY UNUSUAL FEARS? ☐ ☐

122. DO YOU OFTEN HAVE NIGHTMARES? ☐ ☐

123. DO YOU BITE YOUR NAILS? ☐ ☐

124. DO YOU WORRY VERY MUCH? ☐ ☐

125. DO YOU REGARD YOURSELF AS BEING NERVOUS? ☐ ☐

126. HAVE YOU BEEN TREATED OR HOSPITAL-IZED FOR A PSYCHIATRIC ILLESS? ☐ ☐

127. HAVE YOU EVER HAD A NERVOUS BREAKDOWN? ☐ ☐

128. DO YOU HAVE ANY IMPORTANT PROBLEMS IN YOUR HOME LIFE (EG: MARITAL ADJUSTMENT, CHILDREN, IN-LAWS, FINANCES, ETC.)? ☐ ☐

129. ARE THERE ANY SEXUAL MATTERS OR DIFFICULTIES YOU WOULD LIKE TO DISCUSS? ☐ ☐

130. HAVE YOU BEEN MARRIED MORE THAN ONCE? ☐ ☐

131. DO YOU HAVE ANY WORK PROBLEMS WHICH PRODUCE EMOTIONAL STRESS? ☐ ☐

132. DO YOU HAVE UNUSUAL THIRST OR HUNGER? ☐ ☐

(✓)
YES NO

133. DOES A COOL OR WARM ROOM SEEM TO BOTHER YOU MORE THAN FORMERLY, OR MORE THAN IT DOES OTHER PEOPLE? ☐ ☐

134. HAVE YOU EVER BEEN TOLD OF ANY TROUBLE WITH YOUR THYROID GLAND? ☐ ☐

135. HAVE YOU HAD A GOITER? ☐ ☐

136. HAVE YOU NOTICED ANY CHANGE OF ANY SORT IN YOUR SKIN? ☐ ☐

137. DO YOU HAVE A SORE, SCAB OR ULCER ANYWHERE THAT FAILS TO HEAL? ☐ ☐

138. HAS YOUR HAIR BECOME ESPECIALLY DRY OR COARSE? ☐ ☐

139. DO YOU PERSPIRE EXCESSIVELY? ☐ ☐

140. DO YOU HAVE ITCHING? ☐ ☐

141. DO YOU HAVE A SKIN BLEMISH OR MOLE THAT BLEEDS, ITCHES OR WHICH HAS CHANGED IN COLOR, SIZE OR SHAPE? ☐ ☐

142. DO YOU HAVE A PERSISTANT SORE OR ROUGHENED AREA AROUND THE LIPS, OR YOUR MOUTH, OR ON YOUR SKIN? ☐ ☐

143. DO YOU DEVELOP SKIN BRUISES (BLACK AND BLUE MARKS) VERY EASILY AND OFTEN? ☐ ☐

144. DO YOU HAVE A BLEEDING TENDENCY? ☐ ☐

145. HAVE YOU EVER HAD OR BEEN TOLD YOU HAD ANY OF THE FOLLOWING ILLNESSES?

MEASLES ☐ ☐

GERMAN MEASLES ☐ ☐

WHOOPING COUGH ☐ ☐

MUMPS ☐ ☐

HERPES ZOSTER (SHINGLES) ☐ ☐

ENCEPHALITIS (SLEEPING SICKNESS) ☐ ☐

DIPHTHERIA ☐ ☐

POLIOMYELITIS ☐ ☐

TONSILLITIS ☐ ☐

RHEUMATIC FEVER ☐ ☐

ST. VITUS DANCE (CHOREA) ☐ ☐

PLEURISY ☐ ☐

PNEUMONIA ☐ ☐

INFECTIOUS MONONUCLEOSIS ("MONO") ☐ ☐

TUBERCULOSIS ☐ ☐

HEPATITIS-(JAUNDICE) ☐ ☐

TYPHOID FEVER ☐ ☐

AMEBIC DYSENTARY ☐ ☐

TROPICAL DISEASE ☐ ☐

PARASITIC DISEASE-INFECTION ☐ ☐

MALARIA ☐ ☐

HIVES ☐ ☐

HAY FEVER ☐ ☐

ASTHMA ☐ ☐

GOUT ☐ ☐

(✓)
YES NO

145. CONTINUED

	YES	NO
DIABETES	☐	☐
ARTHRITIS	☐	☐
PHLEBITIS (AN INFECTED VEIN)	☐	☐
VARICOSE VEINS	☐	☐
A LUMP, GROWTH, CYST, POLYP, TUMOR, OR CANCER IN ANY LOCATION.	☐	☐

146. HAVE YOU EVER RECEIVED A BLOOD TRANSFUSION? ☐ ☐

147. HAVE YOU EVER HAD **TREATMENT** (NOT EXAMINATION) BY X-RAY OR RADIATION FOR ANY CONDITION? ☐ ☐

148. HAVE YOU EVER HAD ANY BAD EFFECT, OR ALLERGIC REACTION, FROM A MEDICINE OR INJECTION? ☐ ☐

149. HAVE YOU EVER HAD AN UNEXPLAINED PROLONGED FEVER? ☐ ☐

150. HAVE YOU EVER BEEN TOLD YOU HAVE ALLERGIES? ☐ ☐

151. HAVE YOU EVER BEEN INJURED AT WORK? ☐ ☐

152. HAVE YOU EVER RECEIVED COMPENSATION FOR ANY INDUSTRIAL INJURY OR ILLNESS? ☐ ☐

153. HAVE YOU EVER BEEN RESTRICTED IN YOUR WORK OR PHYSICAL ACTIVITY, OR GIVEN LIMITED DUTY IN MILITARY SERVICE BECAUSE OF YOUR HEALTH? ☐ ☐

154. WERE YOU EVER "TURNED DOWN" FOR ANY WORK, OR MILITARY SERVICE, BECAUSE OF YOUR HEALTH? ☐ ☐

155. DID YOU EVER LEAVE A POSITION BECAUSE OF YOUR HEALTH? ☐ ☐

156. HAVE YOU OVER ANY PROLONGED PERIOD BEEN EXPOSED TO EXCESSIVE NOISE, DUST, FUMES OR OTHER CONDITIONS WHICH MIGHT HAVE AN EFFECT ON HEALTH? ☐ ☐

157. WERE YOU EVER REFUSED LIFE INSURANCE OR ASKED TO PAY A HIGHER-THAN-STANDARD PREMIUM? ☐ ☐

158. WERE YOU EVER ON ACTIVE DUTY IN A MILITARY SERVICE? ☐ ☐

159. IF YOU WERE IN A MILITARY SERVICE, WERE YOU GIVEN A DISABILITY RATING WHEN DISCHARGED? ☐ ☐

160. HAVE YOU EVER HAD ANY OF THESE SPECIAL DIAGNOSTIC STUDIES? IF YES, GIVE DATES:

	(✓) YES	NO	DATE(S)
EXERCISE EKG (TREADMILL)	☐	☐	_____
THALLIUM SCAN (HEART)	☐	☐	_____
ECHOCARDIOGRAM	☐	☐	_____
CT SCAN (CAT SCAN)	☐	☐	_____
SIGMOIDOSCOPY	☐	☐	_____
COLONOSCOPY	☐	☐	_____
GLAUCOMA TEST	☐	☐	_____

(✓)
YES NO

161. HAVE YOU EVER HAD ANY ILLNESSES, FRACTURES OR OTHER INJURIES NOT ASKED ABOUT THUS FAR? ☐ ☐

_____
_____
_____
_____
_____
_____
_____
_____
_____
_____
_____
_____
_____
_____
_____
_____
_____
_____
_____

162. APPROXIMATELY HOW MANY DAYS WERE YOU AWAY FROM WORK IN THE PAST YEAR BECAUSE OF ILLNESS OR INJURY? _____

163.

FAMILY HISTORY

RELATIONSHIP	AGE	IF LIVING, STATE OF HEALTH	IF DEAD, AGE AT DEATH AND CAUSE
FATHER			
MOTHER			
☐ BROTHER OR ☐ SISTER			
☐ BROTHER OR ☐ SISTER			
☐ BROTHER OR ☐ SISTER			
☐ BROTHER OR ☐ SISTER			
☐ BROTHER OR ☐ SISTER			
☐ BROTHER OR ☐ SISTER			
MOTHER'S MOTHER			
MOTHER'S FATHER			
FATHER'S MOTHER			
FATHER'S FATHER			
WIFE OR HUSBAND, PRESENT			
WIFE OR HUSBAND, FORMER (IF ANY)			
☐ SON OR ☐ DAUGHTER			
☐ SON OR ☐ DAUGHTER			
☐ SON OR ☐ DAUGHTER			
☐ SON OR ☐ DAUGHTER			
☐ SON OR ☐ DAUGHTER			
☐ SON OR ☐ DAUGHTER			

164. HAVE ANY OF THE PERSONS LISTED ABOVE, OR ANY BLOOD RELATIVE, EVER HAD ANY OF THE FOLLOWING?

	YES	NO	IF YES, STATE RELATIONSHIP
ARTHRITIS OR RHEUMATISM			
ASTHMA, HAY FEVER OR OTHER ALLERGIES			
CANCER			
DIABETES			
HEART TROUBLE			
HIGH BLOOD PRESSURE			
KIDNEY TROUBLE			
DUODENAL OR STOMACH ULCER			
TUBERCULOSIS			
NERVOUS BREAKDOWN OR EMOTIONAL OR MENTAL DISORDER			
EPILEPSY OR CONVULSIVE DISORDER			
BLEEDING TENDENCY			
MISCARRIAGE			
INFANT BORN DEAD, OR DYING AT OR SOON AFTER BIRTH			

165. A. WHAT IS THE MOST YOU HAVE EVER WEIGHED?

———————— LBS.

B. WHAT IS YOUR USUAL WEIGHT?

———————— LBS.

C. WHAT IS YOUR PRESENT WEIGHT?

———————— LBS.

166. PHYSICAL ACTIVITY: WHICH CATEGORY DO YOU FIT IN?

☐ **ACTIVE** - AN ATHLETE IN TRAINING OR A PERSON WHO EXERCISES AT A LEVEL COMPARABLE TO RUNNING AT LEAST 2 MILES; 3 OR MORE DAYS A WEEK.

TYPE OF EXERCISE-

DISTANCE-

TIME-

TIMES/WEEK-

☐ **MODERATELY ACTIVE** - PLANNED RECREATION AT LEAST 3 DAYS PER WEEK, OR INVOLVEMENT IN A HEAVY OCCUPATION SUCH AS A CONSTRUCTION OR FARMING.

☐ **OCCASIONALLY ACTIVE** - RECREATION OR PHYSICAL ACTIVITY LESS THAN 2-3 TIMES PER WEEK.

☐ **SEDENTARY** - ONLY NORMAL DAILY ACTIVITIES SUCH AS EATING, SLEEPING, SITTING, TALKING, A SEDENTARY JOB OR ATTENDING SCHOOL.

167. A. HAVE YOU EVER SMOKED?   ☐ YES ☐ NO

B. HOW MUCH, ON THE AVERAGE DO YOU **NOW** SMOKE?

CIGARETTES PER DAY:————————

CIGARS PER DAY:————————

PIPEFULS PER DAY:————————

C. FOR HOW MANY YEARS ALTOGETHER HAVE YOU, OR DID YOU, SMOKE AN AVERAGE OF:

ONE OR MORE PACKS OF CIGARETTES PER DAY?————————

FIVE OR MORE CIGARS PER DAY? ————————

FIVE OR MORE PIPEFULS OF TOBACCO PER DAY?————————

D. DO, OR DID, YOU INHALE THE SMOKE?   ☐ YES ☐ NO

E. DO YOU USE SNUFF?   ☐ YES ☐ NO
(SMOKELESS TOBACCO PRODUCTS)

168. HOW MUCH OF THE FOLLOWING BEVERAGES DO YOU USUALLY DRINK?

CUPS OF COFFEE PER DAY?————————

CUPS OF TEA PER DAY? ————————

GLASSES OF BEER?

———————— GLASSES PER   ☐ DAY OR ☐ WEEK

GLASSES OF WINE?

———————— GLASSES PER   ☐ DAY OR ☐ WEEK

DRINKS OF WHISKEY, GIN OR SIMILAR LIQUORS?

———————— DRINKS PER   ☐ DAY OR ☐ WEEK

169. INDICATE THE NUMBER WHICH BEST DESCRIBES THE STRESS LEVEL, PRESSURE OR STRAIN IN THE FOLLOWING AREAS OF YOUR LIFE. BASE THE RATING ON 1-10 SCALE; 1. BEING VERY RELAXED AND 10. BEING VERY STRESSFUL.

JOB ————————

HOMELIFE ————————

170. A. HOW MANY WEEKS OF VACATION WERE YOU ENTITLED TO LAST YEAR?

————————

B. HOW MANY WEEKS DID YOU TAKE?————————

171. HOW MANY HOURS OF SLEEP DO YOU AVERAGE PER 24 HOURS?

————————

172. INDICATE APPROXIMATE NUMBER OF HOURS YOU SPEND IN THE AVERAGE **WEEK** DOING THE FOLLOWING AND CHECK HOW MUCH SATISFACTION YOU FEEL YOU GET OUT OF EACH.

ACTIVITY	HOURS	SATISFACTION			
		NONE	LITTLE	MODERATE	MUCH
OVERTIME WORK AT USUAL PLACE OF WORK?					
BUSINESS WORK OR BUSINESS READING DONE AT HOME?					
EVENING CLASSES AND RELATED HOMEWORK?					
WORK ON HOME OR GARDEN?					
HOUSEKEEPING, COOKING, OR CARE OF CHILDREN, ETC.?					
COMMUNITY WORK SUCH AS FOR CHURCH, SCHOOL, SCOUTING, ETC.?					
READING?					
WATCHING TELEVISION?					
HOBBIES OR OTHER DIVERSIONS OR ACTIVITES? (LIST)					

173. INDICATE WHETHER YOU BELIEVE YOUR HEALTH NOW TO BE —

EXCELLENT _____ FAIR _____

GOOD_____ POOR _____

174. WHAT DO **YOU** FEEL IS YOUR PRINCIPAL HEALTH PROBLEM AT THE PRESENT TIME?

_____

_____

_____

_____

_____

175. IS THERE ANYTHING CONCERNING YOUR ☐ YES ☐ NO HEALTH THAT HAS NOT BEEN INCLUDED IN THIS QUESTIONAIRE WHICH YOU WOULD LIKE TO DISCUSS?

_____

_____

_____

_____

_____

176. IMMUNIZATIONS   YEAR

SMALL POX   _____

TETANUS   _____

POLIO — INJ   _____

POLIO — ORAL   _____

CHOLERA   _____

YELLOW FEVER   _____

TYPHOID   _____

OTHER   _____

177. PLEASE INDICATE IF YOU ARE INTERESTED IN:

BREAST SELF EXAMINATION TRAINING ☐

STRESS MANAGEMENT SESSIONS ☐

SMOKING CONTROL SESSIONS ☐

NUTRITION EDUCATION CLASSES ☐

FITNESS LEVEL TESTING ☐

A PLANNED EXERCISE PROGRAM ☐

NAME _____   DATE _____

HX   PMH

SR

	DONE
VISION	
AUDIOMETRY	
STOOLS - OCC. BL.	
URINALYSIS	
EKG	
VITAL CAP.	
BLOOD CHEM.	
PPD.	

S.H. TOBACCO

ALCOHOL

EXERCISE

STRESS LEVEL

DIET

PHYSICAL FINDINGS

1.

2.

3.

4.

RECOMMENDATIONS - CONSULTATIONS, FURTHER TESTS

1. _____

2. _____

3. _____

4. _____

5. _____

6. _____

7. _____

DIAGNOSIS

1.

2.

3.

4.

5.

6.

PHYSICAL EXAMINATION		PULSE	TEMP.	WEIGHT	HEIGHT

GENERAL APPEARANCE

	NORMAL				
BLOOD PRESSURE		NURSE RT / LEFT /		PHYSICIAN RT / LEFT /	
HAIR/SCALP		COLOR TEXTURE		ALOPECIA ERUPTION	
SKULL		TENDERNESS DEFORMITY			
EARS		CANALS DRUMS DISCHARGE TOPHI CERUMEN			
NOSE		TURBINATES SEPTUM DISCHARGE			
SINUSES		FRONTAL MAXILLARY TENDERNESS			
EYES		COLOR CONJUCTIVA SCLERA PTOSIS			
		NYSTAGMUS EXOPHTHALMUS CATARACT			
		PUPILS ROUND REGULAR EQUAL			
		REACT TO LIGHT AND ACCOMMODATION			
FUNDI		DISCS HEMORRHAGE EXUDATE VESSELS			
FACE		SCARS MUSCLE MOVEMENT SENSORY PERCEPTION			
LIPS		CYANOSIS HERPES ULCERS			
MOUTH		BREATH ULCERS ABNORMAL PIGMENTATION LEUKOPLAKIA			
TEETH		CLEAN CARIES CHEWING SURFACE			
		DENTURES- UPPER LOWER PARTIAL COMPLETE			
GUMS		PYORRHEA BLEEDING RECESSION			
TONGUE		MIDLINE PROTRUSION TREMOR LESIONS			
TONSILS		PRESENT INFECTION			
PHARYNX		EXUDATE INJECTION INFECTION			
LARYNX		VOICE NORMAL VOCAL CORDS TRACHEA MIDLINE			
NECK		VEIN CONGESTION NORMAL PULSATION SCARS			
		STIFFNESS BRUIT			
THYROID		MASSES NOT PALP MULTINODULAR			
LYMPH GLANDS		POST CERVICAL ANT. CERVICAL AXILLARY INGUINAL			
SPINE		TENDERNESS R.O.M. CURVATURE			
THORAX		SYMMETRICAL DEFORMITY EQUAL EXPANSION			

RESPIRATORY	REGULAR	DEPTH	SYMMETRICAL		RATE	
LUNGS	PERCUSSION		AUSCULTATION		BREATH SOUNDS	
	VOICE SOUNDS		RALES			
HEART	REGULAR	A-2	P-2		RATE	THRILL
	MURMURS-					
	APEX IMPULSE		ICS			IN TO L. OF MSL
BREASTS	SIZE		MASSES		TENDERNESS	
PULSE	RATE		REGULAR	DEFICIT	VOLUME	
ABDOMEN	SCARS		DILATED VEINS	RIGIDITY	TENDERNESS	
	MUSCLE GUARDING		MASSES		FLUID WAVE	
	BOWEL SOUNDS		LIVER PALPABLE		KIDNEYS PALPABLE	
	SPLEEN PALPABLE		PERISTALSIS		BRUIT	
LEGS	VARICOSITIES		ULCERS	EDEMA	DORSALIS PEDIS PALPABLE	
	ARCHES			R.O.M.		
JOINTS	FINGER JOINT CHANGES			TOE JOINT CHANGES		
ARTERIES	ARTERIOSCLEROTIC					
REFLEXES	PATELLAR	ACHILLES	BICEPS	TRICEPS	EPIGASTRIC	
	CLONUS	BABINSKI	VIBRATION	CREMASTERIC	RHOMBERG	
ARMS/HANDS	CYANOSIS		TREMOR	FINGER CLUBBING	WET PALMS	
GENITALIA	DISCHARGE		ULCERS	EDEMA	LESIONS	
	TESTICLE			VARICOCELE	HYDROCELE	
	VULVA		VAGINA		CERVIX	
	UTERUS		ADENEXA			
INGUINAL	HERNIA		RELAXED RING			
RECTAL	HEMORRHOIDS		MASSES	TENDERNESS	BLOOD	
PROSTATE	ENLARGED		TENDER			
SKIN	TEXTURE		MOISTURE	CYANOSIS	JAUNDICE	
	ERUPTION		LESIONS		ABNORMAL PIGMENTATION	

PHYSICAL EXAM			
PHYSICIAN'S NOTES			

URINALYSIS			
SPECIFIC GRAVITY		BLOOD	
COLOR		PROTEIN	
PH		MICROSCOPIC:	
SUGAR		UROBILINOGEN	
ACETONE		BILIRUBIN	

STOOL-OCCULT BLOOD				SIGMOIDOSCOPY
#1	#2	#3	#4	DISTANCE EXAMINED _____ cm

TONOMETER TEST	WT	READING	MM. OF HG	
RIGHT EYE				
LEFT EYE				

PELVIC EXAM
PAP SMEAR
X-RAYS
PPD

VITAL CAPACITY		
FEV_1		FVC

ENDNOTES

1. Interview with Leo C. Beebe.

CHAPTER 4

HOW MANAGERS AFFECT AND DEAL WITH EMPLOYEE STRESS

Any active life is more or less
stressful, but life's stresses are
not necessarily destructive.
Indeed, the challenge they pose may
open the door to one of life's
greatest joys, savoring the
satisfaction of achievement.[1]
Stewart Wolf

Much has been written on the many ways people cope with stress. Most corporate employee assistance programs include at least one, and often several, stress management programs. Our goal in writing this chapter is not to discuss the numerous traditional strategies for dealing with stress. Rather, we want to share the insights we have gained about management's view of stress within Corporate America and report some of the newer management thinking about stress control and reduction.

STRESS EQUALS $$$

Pity the poor business man. When
the help isn't clamoring for more
pay and shorter hours, the
customers are yelling for lower
prices and better services.

One of the largest and fastest growing expenses facing Corporate America results from employee stress. Workers' compensation claims for stress-related problems have tripled since 1980, and the number of lawsuits based on "stress injuries" has grown dramatically. On April 7, 1988, *The Wall Street Journal*[2] reported that "Psychological disorders have become one of the fastest-growing occupational ills of the decade. Stress now accounts for about 14 percent of occupational-disease claims, up from less than 5 percent in 1980."

In addition, companies are paying millions of dollars for employee stress management programs as well as for the services of psychologists and psychiatrists. *Within the fitness/wellness movement, dealing with stress and stress-related diseases is becoming the number-one issue.*

The problem is complicated by the inability of some employees to recognize the signs indicating they are under excessive stress. Therefore, these employees are less likely to take advantage of company-provided stress reduction and coping programs. This is very unfortunate, since stress may be implicated in illnesses, including coronary artery disease. When a person is under stress, the level of adrenalin and adrenocortical hormones increases, which tends to accelerate the development of coronary artery disease. Stress also causes an increase in blood pressure. These reactions to stress date back to the primitive "flight or fight" syndrome. In earlier times, a person would either fight or flee and, at some point, the fight or the flight would end, the stressor would be removed, and the person's physical system would readjust to a normal level.

In today's society, however, fight or flight from a stressful situation may not be possible. Stress may build and turn into very unhealthy anger and, over time, result in the deterioration of a person's health. Thus, it is important for those in high-stress situations to obtain assistance to reduce their stress levels.

It is a fact of Corporate American life that many employees face high levels of stress resulting from their jobs and/or their personal lives and that the dollar cost of stress to employers is escalating rapidly. Our research would suggest that programs in stress reduction and coping with stress will not only be available to most employees in the future, but also may become mandatory. These programs are likely to be included along with other employee training programs and to be considered a necessary part of every employee's benefits package.

HOW MANAGERS VIEW STRESS

> Automobile-manufacturing tycoon to
> assistant: "If those traffic jams
> didn't cause our workers to be
> late, we could make 200 more cars
> each week."

In asking managers if they thought the level of stress employees face today is greater than in the past, we noted that stress is a relatively new word in our vocabulary. If one looks back only two generations to World War II, stress hardly is mentioned. But those who were under bombardment, as well as those on the battlefields and those left behind at home, must have experienced very high levels of stress. Yet, stress was not a commonly used term, and people did what they had to do to survive. What has changed?

Mr. Carl Sempier, past President of Mannington Resilient Floors,[3] put it this way:

> As a country enters an age where morality declines and the ability to distinguish between right and wrong gets blurred, I think people become vulnerable to a great deal of stress.
>
> We have to understand that we are all faced with stress. How we react to it depends on how secure we are within ourselves and that we know what really matters in our lives, that we have our priorities in pretty good order so that they don't change from day to day and we don't run after other people's goals.
>
> My perception is that there is no more stress in the workplace now than there was yesterday, but there is a heightened awareness of it. As our medical and diagnostic skills have increased, we are now able to relate more illness and other employee problems to being stress related.
>
> Uncertainty and lack of consistency causes stress. Years ago there was uncertainty about coming out of the Depression. Today we have an overwhelming flow of data which can cause stress. Per-

sonal expectations are higher. We have kids with personal schedules that would have paled an adult 20 years ago. All of this adds stress in our lives.

Lack of Predictability and Control as Stressors

One manager we interviewed felt that stress has always existed, but that we know much more about it today and how it relates to health problems. He noted that the "good old days" were really terrible. For example, working conditions were poor, and laborers, frequently accompanied by their children, toiled long hours for low wages. Up until the Civil War, a walk in Washington, D.C., on a rainy day meant you were up to your knees in mud. The Sunbelt was virtually uninhabitable until 20 years ago. Although we have a much better standard of living today than even 20 years ago, we have a much greater degree of unpredictability today than ever before. *Many managers believe that it is this feeling of unpredictability that causes the most stress among employees.*

For example, the downsizing of Corporate America and the elimination of many employees, along with the uncertainty resulting from numerous acquisitions, has led to a very high level of employee insecurity at nearly every tier. Corporate cost-cutting and restructuring actions, which are completely beyond the employees' control and may result in employee termination, were reported as causing extremely high levels of stress.

The following statement, taken from the first quarter 1988 report to shareholders of a billion-dollar consumer products firm, is particularly representative of a stress-inducing situation:

> We cut overhead by eliminating 500 positions in our . . . headquarters. We analyzed our manufacturing capability and made substantial cost savings. Between the end of 1986 and mid-1988, we will have closed 10 production plants, reducing our internal production capacity by 40 percent.

Having a secure job and having some degree of control over the security of the job are very important factors in moderating stress. Managers noted that when takeover rumors ran through the hallways, productivity dropped. Employees hunkered down, focused all their energies on protecting their own interests, tended to make fewer decisions, avoided taking responsibility, and used company time to update their resumes and talk with job recruiters. Even if the takeover rumors were completely untrue and management publicly denied them, many employees still reacted as if a takeover were imminent. Employees distrusted anything senior managers said, believing that the "official story" could change from day to day. One of the authors recalls a telephone conversation with a senior vice president of a major investment firm. Midway through the conversation, the executive suddenly blurted out, "My God, we've just been taken over." He had no idea or advance warning of the takeover. This incident is representative of a widespread sense of uneasiness among employees in many companies and a distrust of senior management as well as of the capitalistic system that permits financiers to play corporate monopoly.

Control, both with respect to job security and the job itself, was reported as being very important to employees. Managers indicate that employees suffered more stress-related problems when they had little control over the pace of the work and the working methods. These observations clearly lend strong support for increasing employee participation through quality circles and similar organizational development programs.

Managers also observe that employees who hold positions with a lot of responsibility but little power suffer from high levels of stress. For example, upper-level managers who have more decision-making power generally seem to suffer from less stress than lower-level managers who have limited decision-making power. When a company takeover is involved and upper-level managers' jobs are at stake, however, they may suffer from very high levels of stress.

Language and Communications Barriers as Stressors

Particularly among immigrants, language barriers and not understanding the job were also noted as stress-producing factors. As more immigrants enter the labor force, management will need to become more cognizant of the special needs of this population so that stress will be minimized and productivity enhanced.

Michael Matteson[4] notes the need for special consideration of stress during the early periods of a person's employment.

For a great many individuals the first few months in a new job with a new organization are particularly stressful as they struggle to learn the ropes, become accepted by others, make a positive contribution to organizational goals and objectives, and, very importantly, come to grips with the inevitable disappointments and gaps between personal expectations and organizational realities. The number and magnitude of such gaps, as well as the individual's ability to adapt, determine in large part the extent to which the individual-organizational marriage will be a successful one or will be marked by frustration and conflict and ultimate divorce.

White-Collar Tools as Stressors

Over and above the problems of job insecurity, language barriers, and lack of involvement in decision making, managers also noted that those tools that so greatly enhance productivity, such as the telephone and the computer, add stress. When the phone rings, it disrupts thinking and produces uncertainty—who is calling and why? This differs significantly from a scheduled appointment, which can be prepared for in advance and therefore can be rendered potentially less stressful.

Similarly, the computer provides information, sometimes at levels greater than can be readily digested, thus causing stress. When the computer system is "down" or malfunctions, an employee may be forced to stop working and consequently falls behind. Such unpredictable circumstances outside of an employee's control can be very stress-producing.

Computer monitoring of phone calls and of persons who work at computer stations were cited as causes of stress, along with poorly designed work areas. For example, glare, extremes in temperature, offensive noise, uncomfortable furniture—all of these can add to stress both in the workplace and at home.

MANAGERS AS STRESS PRODUCERS AND REDUCERS

A modern employer is one who is
looking for people between the ages
of 25 and 30 with 40 years'
experience

When we interviewed corporate executives and members of the medical community, we were surprised to find that many executives have concluded that *a very substantial portion of employee stress was directly related to working for "stressful managers."* These executives told us that they were spending a lot on programs to help employees deal effectively with stress and intended to increase spending on training managers not to be "stressful managers."

A vice president for human resources of a major food corporation provided this insightful commentary on stress:

I think there is more stress today than in the past. It has to do with the rapid change of pace in society today. There is more stimulation in the environment and a greater expectation that you should be able to control it.

The fact that we are expected to make our own decisions earlier in life, construct our own curriculum, and find our own way, somehow leads to the notion that we should have mastery over all these things.

In an agrarian society there was stress, for example, if it didn't rain. The stress was relieved through a religious or other ceremonial activity which acknowledged that things were beyond our control. Once you performed that activity you basically left it in God's hands and forgot about it.

Religion is being replaced by a sense of something called spirituality. Organized religion provides real answers—spirituality does not. With the advent of spirituality, there is a real expectation in many peoples' minds that they should be able to handle all of the decision-making themselves. This adds stress to their lives.

Family life used to be simpler. Business is more complicated and changeable. We demand more from the workers and throw more information and technology at them. The only thing that doesn't change is change. People can become really overloaded from it.

Accounting can be an especially stressful profession, particularly during tax season. We asked William Spencer, National Director of Human Resources at Laventhol and Horwath, how his firm deals with stress and stress management.[5]

> Predictability is important for employees, but there is some lack of predictability in all organizations. Everyone wants growth—individual, personal, and financial. We all espouse that. Yet, in a metaphysical sense we can't have growth without change, and change inevitably produces stress.
>
> Stress is generated internally from external stimuli. We can help our people by teaching our managers to use people more effectively. For example, our deadlines are our clients' deadlines. If a deadline is not achievable, we should tell the client straight out, rather than make a commitment that we know we cannot honor. That would help to relieve our employees of stress.
>
> We can help reduce stress by providing sound leadership that better understands stress. It is our job to make our line managers more effective. We try to teach our managers in the vital importance of employee evaluations in providing a surprise-free atmosphere. Performance evaluation can be very effective in reducing stress. People want to know where they stand and don't like surprises!
>
> I feel it is better to invest money in training managers to be better managers and thereby lessen employee stress than to invest money in psychologists' bills for employees.

William M. Kizer, Chairman and CEO of Central States Health & Life Co.,[6] noted that stress can be good or bad. If the stress encourages and motivates us, it is called euphoric stress or "eustress." He noted that management's responsibility is to turn harmful stress to eustress by helping employees take charge of their own health and by providing training so that employees can do their jobs more effectively.

The vice president for human resources of a major food corporation quoted earlier also noted that it is important that managers ask themselves if they are doing certain activities that may cause stress and, if so, what they can do to control it:

> I think there are ways we can handle employee stress. Employee participation gives people more of a sense of control and is positive

if managed correctly. We are not trying to be paternalistic and say that we want to solve the employee's problems. Rather, our challenge is to try to give the employee some means of coping with stress when he or she is ready for it. This kind of thinking must replace the paternalistic idea that we know what is best for the employee.

It is important to try to change managers to become less stress producing. But you can't expect to change every manager. Some managers can learn to change a great deal, others much less. We therefore have to realize that many employees will be subjected to a lot of stress because of a particular boss's management style.

Mr. Sempier remarked that if you are in a management role where there is uncertainty, or people around you are not sure of their roles, or if you work under a highly emotional manager who eventually is going to blow up, all of this causes stress over and beyond any considerations of the actual job to be accomplished. In other words, *stressful people cause stress.*

He noted that Mannington Mills has a supervisory training program that can be tailored to meet an individual's particular needs. The company's stress programs emphasize that people need to become aware of stressful situations so they can plan to deal with them before physical or emotional damage results.

Bertram Dinman[7] provides an excellent summary of what management can do to be most effective in minimizing on-the-job stress:

> Management is most effective when corporate objectives are made clear, when job designs are coherent and logical, when relationships among coworkers and with supervisors are clearly delineated, and when limitations on freedom to act on individual initiative are explicit.
>
> On the other hand, when the job specification is vague, when there is ambiguity as to functional and administrative accountability, when productivity demands are unrealistic, or when responsibility is maximized in the face of little authority, stress responses among workers may ensue. Thus, failure to communicate can lead to avoidable impairments of performance and even of health of employees.

JOBS AS STRESS PRODUCERS:
A CAUTIONARY NOTE

> It is not work that kills people;
> it is worry. Work is healthy; you
> can hardly put more upon people
> than they can bear. Worry is rust
> upon the blade. It is not the
> revolution that destroys the
> machinery, but the friction.
> *Henry Ward Beecher*

In our research, we reviewed articles listing such "stressful" jobs as policemen and air traffic controllers. As noted earlier, jobs entailing a lot of responsibility but little authority seem to be more stress-producing. Ronald Burke[8] comments that to some degree, however, the actual level of stress may be more of a "self-fulfilling prophecy," where the employees "begin to believe their own myth." He cites studies of air traffic controllers and notes that during interviews,

> They often commented that they had been told so often that their job was expected to have such severe negative consequences on their health and home-life and that they would "burn out" at an early age, that they began looking for these problems where they might not otherwise have existed. Furthermore, they frequently complained about the pressure and frustration of having others around them also expecting and looking for signs in them of the inevitable deterioration and breakdown.[9]

People do tend to believe what they are told, even when the person making the statement has little or no knowledge of the facts. They focus on and look forward to the fulfillment of prophecies. Thus, a person who is told that he or she is in a high stress job may start looking for signs of stress and actually exhibit physical symptoms in order to let the prophecy self-fulfill. This kind of response is noted by Bernie Siegel, M.D.:[10]

> The physician's habitual prognosis of how much time a patient has left is a terrible mistake. It's a self-fulfilling prophecy. It must be

resisted even though many patients keep asking "How long? How long?" They want someone else to define the limits of life instead of taking part in the determination themselves. People who like their doctors and who are passive often die right on schedule, as though to prove them right.

These observations suggest that rather than management simply talking about stress as "a problem," per se, management should try to reduce job stress, assist employees in reducing personal stresses, and focus on the positive, healthy aspects of the job and work environment.

THE SYNERGISM OF STRESS

When we wake before morning's
earliest light, little
problems often take on large
proportions and add upon one
another yielding totals more
than we can bear.

The managers and members of the medical community we talked with indicated that stresses from all sources are cumulative in some additive or synergistic way and tend to produce a combined total stress effect on the individual. The two types of job-related stress, those resulting from the physical conditions and those resulting from psychological factors, combine with personal stress to provide a total stress "environment" for each person. Moreover, there appears to be a spillover effect from work to home, leading to domestic tensions. These home stresses are then brought back to the workplace and affect employee performance.

Stress Overload

Our research indicates that no one really understands how these various stresses add together. What's more, few overt signs of cumulating stress may be evident until a person reaches an "overload" condition. The fact that a person who is having to deal with increasing degrees of stress may not exhibit many overt, but rather only subtle, signs of the stress, appears to be an important point in the literature on stress. For senior managers, this implies that *managers should try to become aware of the subtle indications of stress so that appropriate action can be taken before a person experiences overload and suffers health or other stress-related problems.*

At what point this overload is actually reached varies greatly among individuals. For example, a person may be able to deal with the stress of job insecurity by itself; however, if a stressful personal situation, such as the closing of a day care center or the need to care for a sick parent, is added to the stress of an insecure job, then he or she may not be able to handle all of the stress taken together.

It is not clear why some set of conditions or events will produce a stressful reaction in some people and not in others. The situation may be analogous to the medical interactions described by Dr. Frankl in the Medical Component at the end of the book. He notes that if a person is a cigarette smoker, he or she is more likely to contract lung cancer. But some people who smoke two packs a day never contract the disease. Is there a direct cause and effect link between smoking and contracting cancer? Probably so. But the link between an offending agent such as stress and the development of a health problem involves intermediary processes in biochemistry and genetics that are imperfectly understood at this time. Consequently, *managers should be alert to the subtle changes exhibited by many people under stress and help the individual to reduce the stress or learn how to cope with it before overload takes place.*

Stress overload can lead to a host of physical health problems, in addition to problems such as an inability to concentrate on the job. All of these directly affect the employee's productivity and the employer's bottom line. Therefore, from a management perspective, it makes good sense for companies to provide programs and facilities to help employees to deal with potential personal stress-producing situations, as well as those in the workplace. Thus, as noted in Chapter 1, companies will increasingly have to make accommodations for workers, such as providing on-site day care centers and flexible hours.

During our research we also found that some firms already

have very broad stress-reduction programs and offer specific courses in such subjects as coping with dependent parents or single parenting. The fact that workplace and personal stresses are additive means that companies must address both sources and help employees to cope with both effectively. Appendix A to this chapter includes a self-scoring questionnaire on stress in the job and home/family setting. It provides a useful way to measure stress in these two important environments.

Adding to Stress: Short Vacations, Overtime, Rotating Shifts

In our research, we also found that some managers believe that a person's ability to deal effectively with stress can be enhanced by taking vacations for an extended period, such as two or more consecutive weeks, as opposed to taking every Friday off during the summer. Being away from the job for two or more weeks appears to give the person time to "recover" from the stress and somehow seems to reduce the synergism which takes place when people are simultaneously placed under stress from a variety of sources. If these observations are correct, then companies may want to consider policies which would require employees to take longer vacations rather than take their vacations in piecemeal fashion.

Managers also noted increased irritability (a sign of stress) exhibited by workers who worked overtime. It appears that regular leisure time is important to maintaining reduced stress levels. Working additional hours obviously intrudes upon this leisure time. Therefore, managers will want to consider the use of overtime very judiciously. In addition, managers should consider the use of four-day workweeks with three-day breaks. Finally, we noted that some managers were considering more off-hour recreational activities for employees and their families.

With the introduction of high-technology equipment, many companies have increased the use of shift work. But working second or third shifts tends to interfere with normal body rhythms and thereby disrupts sleep patterns. For some people the problem is especially pronounced if they do not have access to a quiet room for sleeping during the day. *Managers report increasing degrees of stress-related problems when people work rotating shifts.* Managers, therefore, should consider ways to avoid rotating shifts, perhaps by using some wage inducement to encourage employees to work second or third shift on a permanent basis.

During our discussions with managers, we noted an increased awareness of what causes on-the-job stress and personal stress. Many managers also believe that stress accounts for increased costs to the company in absenteeism and medical expenses. This heightened awareness is leading managers to examine carefully all aspects of the work and the work environment to help reduce stress.

We anticipate many new and perhaps novel ideas will emerge as a consequence of the very high dollar cost of stress. They will likely represent significant departures from the more traditional employee assistance programs, which tend to focus more on helping the employee deal with stress than preventing it. These programs tend to view stress as a "disease" to be treated. The more practical approach, logically, is not to acquire the disease in the first place. This means providing a physical and psychological work environment that minimizes stress and helping employees to eliminate stressful problems in their personal lives. Measures taken to minimize workplace and personal stress are likely to be less expensive and more effective than coping programs and psychologists' services.

HOW MANAGERS ARE HANDLING THEIR OWN STRESS

To be free of stress is to be dead.[11]
E. M. Gherman, M.D.

Although managers were usually very willing to discuss the problems and costs of stress, along with the ways their companies were dealing with stress, most were reluctant to discuss stress in their own lives. We were fortunate that a number of managers (who asked to remain anonymous) were willing to share some of their personal experiences and feelings about their own stress.

Before we share their feelings with you, we would like to emphasize the problem of stress within the managerial ranks by means
of a quote from *The Wall Street Journal.*[12]

> All across the country this stress is building among middle man-
> agers, the junior officers and senior NCOs of the American business
> army. It is harming them physically, emotionally and mentally. And
> while their corporate employers may be leaner—they are certainly
> meaner—it's clear that the increased pressure they're putting on
> middle managers is frequently impairing performance instead of
> stimulating it. Working scared and tired, many managers simply
> aren't working well, and confess that their zeal and loyalty to their
> companies is crumbling.

One manager we talked with told us of his uneasiness about
using the company's stress management programs. His feeling
(which may be groundless) was that top management viewed them
as something for the lower-level employees who couldn't keep it all
together without outside help. Although he said that he was feeling very stressed in his job, he didn't feel comfortable with the
idea of participating in one of the company-sponsored programs.
He had considered seeing a psychologist, but felt that he could not
personally afford the services and was fearful of submitting the
bills to his employer, even though his employer's medical coverage
included partial reimbursement for psychotherapy.

A young female manager described her irritable stomach and
the need to take antacids on a regular basis following her promotion. She said that she felt competent to do the job and that her
initial reviews were positive. She felt, however, that her contemporaries, most of whom were men, viewed her with some disdain
and had not accepted her as a person. She was very uncomfortable
in the position but was reluctant to discuss the matter with her
supervisor for fear that he would think that she was "imagining
things." She indicated plans to consult with a psychologist.

A younger manager described how miserable his life had
been while reporting to an "autocratic" manager who, after a
slight shove out the door, finally retired. His former manager actually boasted about the number of supervisory training and human relations courses and seminars he had attended and had
numerous certificates plastered on his office walls to make the
point. The young manager told us that he had considered leaving

the company but was fearful that he would not get a good recommendation from his boss and so elected to stick it out with the hope that the situation might change. He also told us that during this period he had separated from his wife and was now undergoing marriage counseling with her.

A middle-aged manager described his chronic inability to get along with his subordinates, even though they always achieved their quota. He also told us that there were many transfers within his department; people always coming and going. He attended a series of management workshops which helped him to realize that he was the source of the problem. Once he realized this, he was able to work with the human resources department on a program of management skills tailor-made for him. Now, a year after starting this program, he not only felt much better about himself, but he also had actually started to socialize with his subordinates and was receiving fewer requests for transfers.

An older manager, who had a long service record with his employer, had survived a takeover and two reorganizations. He was retained at no cut in salary, but his duties were increased and his staff reduced. The only "light at the end of the tunnel" was the prospect of early retirement. He was literally wishing his life away and did not feel that any of the stress reduction programs his company offered would be helpful. In addition, he said that he did not have the time to attend them.

From these candid discussions, we came away with the impression that many companies still have a long way to go in reducing on-the-job stress and helping managers and employees to deal with stress. It seems clear, however, that with the escalating cost of stress-related health care, companies will continue to look much more closely at stress and ways to reduce it.

WHAT'S AHEAD?

In Chapter 5 we examine the various ways companies are delivering their fitness and employee assistance programs to employees. Several different approaches are described, each of which has particular advantages, depending on the size and structure of the company.

APPENDIX A

SELF-SCORING JOB AND HOME/FAMILY SETTING STRESS QUESTIONNAIRE[13]

I. STRESS IN THE JOB SETTING

There are 20 questions in this section that attempt to cover, as briefly as possible, the major potential causes of personal stress in the job setting.

The scoring is quite simple. Each question is answered with one answer ranging from A to E. Each answer is translated into points: A = 5; B = 4; C = 3; D = 2; E = 1. By adding up the points for each answer, a total score will be created for this section. The score for this section ranges from a low of 20 points to a high of 85 points, assuming all 20 questions are answered. Cut-off points for stress levels in the Job Setting section are:

Point Range	Stress Level
20 to 48	Low
49 to 76	Medium
77 to 100	High

Stress in the Job Setting

Occupational stress comes from a variety of sources in the workplace. Physical environment, job requirements, co-workers and expectations are a few examples. Read each statement and decide how often it applies to you and your work.

	Almost Always	Frequently	Occasionally	Very Seldom	Never
1. I feel the work I do is boring.	A	B	C	D	E
2. I experience a lot of stress on my job.	A	B	C	D	E
3. Changes in my job situation are threatening to me.	A	B	C	D	E
4. I am quick tempered on my job.	A	B	C	D	E
5. I feel powerless and overburdened in my job.	A	B	C	D	E
6. I am impatient with people I work with who speak slowly or belabor a point.	A	B	C	D	E
7. I am concerned about how well I make decisions at work.	A	B	C	D	E

Stress in the Job Setting (*concluded*)

	Almost Always	Frequently	Occasionally	Very Seldom	Never
8. I feel the people I work with don't like me.	(A)	(B)	(C)	(D)	(E)
9. I become furious when people I work with criticize me in front of others.	(A)	(B)	(C)	(D)	(E)
10. I hurry to get things done at work even when it is not necessary.	(A)	(B)	(C)	(D)	(E)
11. I spend more time working than my job requires.	(A)	(B)	(C)	(D)	(E)
12. My job requires more time than I feel comfortable giving.	(A)	(B)	(C)	(D)	(E)
13. The thought of not having work to do scares me.	(A)	(B)	(C)	(D)	(E)
14. I feel that I have too much responsibility at work.	(A)	(B)	(C)	(D)	(E)
15. I have to be the best at what I do.	(A)	(B)	(C)	(D)	(E)
16. The people I work with are uncooperative and unresponsive.	(A)	(B)	(C)	(D)	(E)
17. My job responsibilities are unclear to me.	(A)	(B)	(C)	(D)	(E)
18. It is unclear to me how others view the quality of my work.	(A)	(B)	(C)	(D)	(E)
19. I feel that my work environment is noisy and uncomfortable.	(A)	(B)	(C)	(D)	(E)
20. Success in my job is the most important thing in my life.	(A)	(B)	(C)	(D)	(E)

II. STRESS IN THE HOME/FAMILY SETTING

The scoring for this section is similar to the Job Setting section. There are 17 questions in the Home/Family section. Each question has an answer ranging from 1 to 5 in point value. The score for this section ranges from a low of 17 points to a high of 85 points, assuming all 17 questions are answered. Cut-off points for stress levels in the Home/Family section are:

Point Range	*Stress Level*
17 to 41	Low
42 to 65	Medium
66 to 85	High

Stress in the Home/Family Setting

Every family has some difficulties that can cause distress from time to time. Read each statement and decide how often it applies to you and your family.

	Almost Always	Frequently	Occasionally	Very Seldom	Never
21. My family does not understand my work commitment.	(A)	(B)	(C)	(D)	(E)
22. I become angry when I cannot control things in my personal life.	(A)	(B)	(C)	(D)	(E)
23. I feel there is never enough time to get things done at home.	(A)	(B)	(C)	(D)	(E)
24. People in my family tell me that I eat too fast.	(A)	(B)	(C)	(D)	(E)
25. I feel infuriated with people close to me.	(A)	(B)	(C)	(D)	(E)
26. I experience a lot of stress in my home and family life.	(A)	(B)	(C)	(D)	(E)
27. I worry about not being able to pay my bills.	(A)	(B)	(C)	(D)	(E)
28. I worry about those close to me dying.	(A)	(B)	(C)	(D)	(E)
29. I am concerned about my relationships with those close to me.	(A)	(B)	(C)	(D)	(E)
30. I worry about my home and family responsibilities.	(A)	(B)	(C)	(D)	(E)
31. I am concerned about my lack of privacy at home.	(A)	(B)	(C)	(D)	(E)
32. Family celebrations are difficult times for me.	(A)	(B)	(C)	(D)	(E)
33. My family does not understand me.	(A)	(B)	(C)	(D)	(E)
34. Members of my family argue.	(A)	(B)	(C)	(D)	(E)
35. I feel depressed and very sad.	(A)	(B)	(C)	(D)	(E)
36. I am uncomfortable with my living situation.	(A)	(B)	(C)	(D)	(E)
37. I am very concerned about the health of a family member.	(A)	(B)	(C)	(D)	(E)

ENDNOTES

1. Stewart Wolf, "Perspective and Preventive Strategies," in *Occupational Stress: Health and Performance at Work*, edited by Stewart Wolf, M.D. and Albert J. Finestone, M.D. (Littleton, MA: PSG Publishing Company, 1986), pp. 136–37.

2. Michael J. McCarthy, "Stressed Employees Look for Relief in Worker's Compensation Claims," *The Wall Street Journal*, April 7, 1988.

3. Interview with Carl G. Sempier.

4. Michael T. Matteson, "Individual-Organizational Relationships: Implications for Preventing Job Stress and Burnout," in *Work Stress: Health Care Systems in the Workplace*, edited by James C. Quick and others (New York: Praeger Publishers, 1987), pp. 162–63.

5. Interview with William E. Spencer.

6. Interview with William M. Kizer.

7. Bertram D. Dinman, "Interactions and Shared Responsibilities of Management, Medical Department, and Employees," in *Occupational Stress: Health and Performance at Work*, pp. 136–37.

8. Ronald J. Burke, "Issues and Implications for Health Care Delivery Systems: A Canadian Approach," in *Work Stress: Health Care Systems In The Workplace*, pp. 42–43.

9. Ibid.

10. Bernie S. Siegel, M.D. *Love, Medicine and Miracles* (New York: Harper & Row, 1986), p. 39.

11. E. M. Gherman, M.D., *Stress and the Bottom Line: A Guide to Personal Well-Being and Corporate Health* (New York: AMACOM, 1981).

12. Amanda Bennett, "Is Your Job Making You Sick?" *The Wall Street Journal*, April 22, 1988, sec. 3, p. 1.

13. Provided by Dr. James C. Gillis, President and CEO, Lifestyle Management Reports, Inc., 368 Congress Street, Boston, MA 02210 (617-451-0440).

CHAPTER 5

DELIVERING FITNESS/ WELLNESS PROGRAMS: A MANAGERIAL PERSPECTIVE

There is this difference between
the two temporal blessings—
health and money; money is the most
envied, but the least enjoyed;
health is the most enjoyed, but the
least envied; and this superiority
of the latter is still more obvious
when we reflect that the poorest
man would not part with health for
money, but that the richest would
gladly part with all his money for
health.
Charles C. Colton

The selection of a particular fitness/wellness program depends primarily on what management wants to accomplish. Programs can be simple or extensive, available on-site or off-site, and may or may not involve physical facilities. For example, Air Products and Chemicals, Inc. (see Section II for a description of their program) has established the following set of goals for their fitness/wellness programs:

- Promoting health.
- Improving better integration of employees at all levels.
- Providing a valid employee recruitment and retention tool.

- Improving quality of work life.
- Making a statement of company values.

Their goals are extensive and capture about as broad a set of objectives as we have seen. On the other hand, other companies might not be interested in utilizing a fitness/wellness program for retention and recruitment purposes. These companies likely would not want to have an on-site fitness center.

The comprehensive Conoco Health and Fitness Program (see Section II for a description of their program) emphasizes such basic behavioral changes as smoking cessation, weight management, and exercise adherence. The program is also an integral part of the Company's concern for a broader range of issues concerning the work environment. These include clean air, pleasant working surroundings, comfortable and functional office furniture and work stations, work/home proximities, and supervisor/subordinate relationships.

From our research, we found that most managers approach the fitness/wellness movement pragmatically. In general, they express these primary interests:

Reducing (or containing) medical costs and minimizing absenteeism.

Increasing the esprit de corps.

Providing a positive company image to the employees, customers, and community as a whole.

Since the primary goal of a fitness/wellness program for most companies is to reduce or contain health-related costs, many have started with a medical or wellness component, and within this component, have looked for areas in which an employee can exercise personal control or responsibility. Smoking ranks first because it is the number-one risk factor in coronary artery disease (which is the number-one killer) and the major contributor to lung and respiratory disease. For this reason, we have chosen to use a comprehensive smoking cessation program as an example of the many ways that wellness programs can be delivered and the philosophy underlying the actual delivery system.

SMOKING CESSATION PROGRAMS

Walking hand in hand with
death assures a speedy
arrival.

Most medical directors agree that getting people to stop smoking
will provide greater bottom-line impact than any other single
wellness program area. What do you do to get people to stop
smoking? Consider the following nine steps designed to set the
stage for a smoking cessation program and to get the employee's
attention:

1. *Strongly encourage senior managers especially to stop
smoking* if any still do. This sets a climate of nonsmoking for the
organization. Establishing the proper corporate climate is essential to the success of any wellness program.

At Greyhound, for example, employees are encouraged to
climb stairs as part of their exercise program. Each morning,
Chairman Teets climbs the 19 flights to his office. (In their
correspondence with us they did not indicate any plans to move
to a taller building.)

Although climbing 19 floors may seem a bit strenuous, some
companies are now encouraging employees to wear exercise
shoes to work so that walking and stair climbing will be more
comfortable. This represents a significant break from the traditional wing-tip shoe, but is a very visible and practical way to
help establish an exercise-oriented corporate culture.

Similarly, if a company wants employees to "eat right," it
must provide low calorie, low cholesterol, and low sodium
choices in its cafeterias. In fact, some company cafeteria menus
indicate caloric, cholesterol, and sodium contents of foods.

2. *Establish a corporate smoking policy* that makes it difficult for people to smoke at work and especially difficult for
people to smoke around others. Recall that passive smoking
(being in the presence of others who are smoking) is almost as
dangerous as active smoking. Be sure to remove ashtrays from

all common areas and post "no smoking" signs conspicuously throughout the facility.

3. *Establish a clean air policy* within the facility. You cannot expect employees to stop smoking if they are (or think they are) exposed to chemical vapors, "dirty" air, fumes, or any other form of pollutants.

4. *Remove all cigarette vending machines from the premises.* Replace these with vending machines offering *wholesome* snack foods.

5. *Display "smoking hazard information" materials,* available from organizations such as the local branch of the American Heart Association or the American Lung Association.

6. *Use the internal house organs, posters, theme contents* and other media to enhance camaraderie and employee identification with company programs.

7. *Get the nonsmoking message into the employees' homes* by means of paycheck envelope stuffers (or other communications techniques). Note that about two thirds of corporate medical claims originate from employees' families, and so it is just as important to get spouses and other family members to stop smoking as it is for the smoking employee.

8. *Have each employee fill out a medical background statement,* such as the one used by Hershey Foods Company and included in Chapter 3. Then, follow up with a report to each employee indicating the risk he or she is taking by smoking.

Many companies use a health profile based on an employee's heredity and lifestyle. The idea, of course, is to attract the employee's attention and interest and to encourage motivation to want to change poor health habits. After all, if an employee is not motivated to change, the likelihood is very small that behavior will be changed.

9. *Consider offering reduced insurance deductibles and copayments* for employees who don't smoke, keep their weight within certain limits, wear seat belts regularly, and meet other appropriate wellness criteria. Money does motivate in many cases. This may also be the time to issue annual "employee compensation statements" showing how much the employer pays for medical costs, FICA, retirement, and other benefits in addition to regular salaries and wages.

When the corporate "no smoking" culture is established, and employees, spouses and family members who smoke are aware of the potential hazards of smoking, and all smokers hopefully are motivated to give up the habit, then it is time to decide what type(s) of smoking cessation programs to use and when to offer them and to whom.

Since most companies do not employ experts on smoking cessation, the services of the American Heart Association, the American Lung Association, the American Cancer Society, or a commercial vendor are frequently used. The actual choice depends on what services are locally available, their cost, and track records. One program is unlikely to work for all employees; consequently, many companies use several. Frequently, companies also reimburse tuition costs for noncompany-sponsored programs, which can even include hypnosis in some cases!

Many companies offer smoking cessation and similar programs during lunch hours and after work. Attendance may be enhanced by offering a program on company time. Daytime programs are usually fine for employees but may be inconvenient for other family members who should also be included. Therefore, evening programs may have to be offered and some incentive given for attending—at least a very cordial atmosphere with beverages (including decaffeinated ones) and a "healthful" snack.

Although smoking cessation programs are frequently offered on a regular basis, some companies take advantage of the promotional opportunities afforded such programs during "The Great American Smokeout" or "Heart Month."

Another important consideration is whether to use an internal medical staff or an external team for the physical examination and health/lifestyle risk analysis. This choice generally depends on the size of the company or facility. Smaller companies may not be able to afford full-time physicians and other medical staff and will have to contract for these services.

Now comes the reward. Employees and family members have kicked the habit. Reward them with "I kicked the habit and feel great" T-shirts and also put their pictures, with stories, in the company newsletter or post them on the bulletin board. *Anyone who stops smoking, loses weight, or reduces cholesterol deserves recognition.*

From this discussion of smoking cessation, you can see the importance of providing a supportive environment that, in effect, says to the employee, "We do what we preach." Indeed, establishing the corporate climate and providing an atmosphere which discourages smoking and encourages wellness are likely to be more important than the actual program.

EMPLOYEE ASSISTANCE PROGRAMS AND BEYOND

Part of the mind's effect on health is
direct and conscious. The extent to which we
love ourselves determines whether we eat
right, get enough sleep, wear seat belts,
exercise, and so on. Each of these choices
is a statement of how much we care about
living. These decisions control about 90
percent of the factors that determine our
state of health.
Bernie S. Siegel, M.D.[1]

Within the general rubric of employee assistance programs, companies we surveyed offer a great variety of programs, services and counseling. Ford Motor Company, for example, indicates the scope typical of many programs, namely, ". . . to help employees resolve existing personal and health problems (employee assistance) and to avoid potential problems through lifestyle modification (health promotion). (See Section II for a complete description of Ford's program.)

The philosophy behind the health management program at Kimberly-Clark centers on ". . . accessible and cost-effective health screening, limited primary care, exercise programs, nursing services, and an employee assistance program. . . ." The idea is that "well-informed, healthy employees are happier, safer, more productive, have less absenteeism, and are more likely to have lower health care costs." (See Section II for a complete description of Kimberly-Clark's program.)

EAP Provider Agencies and Systems

Nearly all of the various EAPs are available from outside agencies or vendors, including, in some cases, those of a medical nature. Frequently, medical services are provided by in-house personnel or a local hospital. In order to maintain confidentiality, most of the counseling programs are offered by outside providers. Companies frequently provide their employees with an 800 number for contacting crisis-intervention counselors, who usually are available round-the-clock. Follow-up counseling with local professionals is also available.

Some of the agencies that companies use to provide programs and services are listed below:

- American Heart Association.
- American Cancer Society.
- American Lung Association.
- YMCA.
- American Red Cross.
- March of Dimes.
- American Health Foundation.
- Cocaine Anonymous.
- Alcoholics Anonymous.
- Narcotics Anonymous.
- Local Hospitals.
- Local Colleges.

At Eastman Kodak (see Section II for a description of their program), some 20 "Occupational Health and Safety Teams" are available, consisting of a Kodak physician, at least one registered nurse, and support personnel from their Safety and Administration Services area. These teams provide many of the medical functions within their EAPs.

Some companies are now employing counselors with master's degrees in social work to provide in-house, confidential counseling. Others are providing their employees with video-cassette libraries on such EAP topics as personal financial planning and stress management.

At L. L. Bean (see Section II for a description of their program), Health and Fitness is being integrated with Occupational Health and Safety. The staffs work together in promoting and administering health risk appraisals, as well as in hypertension screening and follow-up, in teaching work station adjustments and exercises to individual departments, in combining "back schools" with health and fitness program classes, and in helping rehabilitate injured workers.

EAP Programs, Services, and Counseling

Some of the *numerous* programs, services, and counseling programs offered as a part of EAPs are listed below:

- AIDS screening.
- Alcohol and other substance abuse and chemical dependency.
- Back care. This is becoming increasingly more important, as back injuries are very common and often can be avoided by using correct lifting techniques as well as stretching and warm up exercises.
- Blood pressure monitoring. More companies are locating blood pressure machines in high-traffic areas to encourage employees to take their own blood pressure frequently. Sometimes vending machines offering wholesome snacks are placed next to these machines.
- Cancer screening (breast, lung, skin, colorectal, prostate, uterine, and testicular). Some companies also offer on-site mammography.
- Care of the elderly.
- CPR.
- Diabetes testing.
- First aid.
- Grief and loss.
- Hearing care.
- Housing.
- Legal counseling.

- Menopause.
- Off-the-job safety and accident prevention.
- Osteoporosis.
- Parenting, baby and child care. Some companies offer special courses in single parenting.
- Personal financial management. Many companies offer personal financial services to executives. This perk is now filtering down to other employees.
- Personal nutrition and weight control. These programs may include diet programs in addition to courses in understanding food labeling, taking vitamins, healthy cooking, proper microwave cooking, and the nutritional values of fast foods.
- Physical abuse.
- Posture evaluation.
- Premenstrual syndrome.
- Prenatal care.
- Preparation for retirement.
- Prudent consumerism.
- Self-defense and karate. Some companies also offer special courses in self-defense and rape prevention for women.
- Separation and divorce.
- Sexual harassment.
- Stress management. There are a great variety of stress management programs, including such topics as relaxation, yoga, meditation, and dealing with teenagers and sick parents.
- Suicide awareness.
- Tenants' rights.
- Vision testing and glaucoma checks.

Typical of some of the programs offered, we find these available over a two-month period at Warner-Lambert: "Computing Your Nutritional Condition," "How to Have a Healthy Baby," "Take This Job and Shove It" (a three-part workshop designed to help you avoid conflicts and stressful situations), "Relax at Lunch," "Bottoms Up" (facts about constipation, laxatives, and hemorrhoids), "Healthy Meals from a Microwave," "Stressed about Money," "Phobias," "Considering a Vegetarian Diet," "Maximizing Your Nutrition Shopping $$$$," and "Dealing with Disagreements and Conflicts."

EAP Program Utilization

The following breakdown for Eastman Kodak (see Section II for a description of their program) shows the percentage of their EAP caseloads for short-term counseling, assessment, referral and follow-up for employees and families:

> 20 percent substance abuse.
>
> 30 percent professional, legal, and financial assistance.
>
> 50 percent family, marital, and emotional problems.

EXERCISE AND FITNESS PROGRAMS

> There is no economy in going to
> bed early to save candles if the
> result is twins.
> *Chinese proverb*

The primary goal of exercise and fitness programs is to get people to exercise regularly and especially to make regular exercise more attractive to those who do not presently exercise on a regular basis. Other commonly stated goals of fitness programs, and especially programs with on-site fitness centers, include recruitment and retention of employees and providing evidence of a "caring" management.

The Medical Aspects

As Dr. Frankl notes in the Medical Component at the end of the book, the individual employee's physical condition must be clearly established before any exercise program is recommended. Pfizer (see Section II for a description of their program) takes this approach:

> After completing the comprehensive physical, the member has an individualized program orientation. This orientation reviews all test results, previews program involvement and discusses risk factor management. From this point the member proceeds into one of several recommended program tracks.

Asymptomatic healthy individuals with low to moderate risk factors enter the regular program. Individuals with moderate to severe risk factors, hypertension, cardiovascular disease or orthopedic problems are entered into a program or a combination of programs, to provide greater supervision and direction, with more frequent re-testing. Members who scored poorly on their nutritional assessments, are overweight, have poor blood lipid profiles or have health conditions that are in part managed by diet (diabetes, gout, cardiovascular disease, etc.) are assigned to the Nutritional Management Program.

Individuals with documented cardiovascular disease, history of cardiovascular complications or excessive risk factor profiles are entered into the Cardiac Rehabilitation Program. These members are monitored by telemetry while exercising and receive additional counseling on risk factor reduction. Stress testing and other tests relative to their condition will be performed every one to three months as indicated. Members with chronic or acute orthopedic problems are referred to the Orthopedic Rehabilitation Program. These members receive frequent testing and individualized training and if indicated, may undergo treatment with one or more therapeutic modalities.

Hypertensive members are assigned to the Hypertension Intervention group. These members have their blood pressure checked daily and receive further consultation concerning medication, diet, weight reduction, and stress management.

Given the numerous medical implications and ramifications of entering an exercise program, a company certainly doesn't want to give anyone a free membership to the local YMCA or health club or even encourage people to climb stairs without first assessing each employee's physical condition. *Before anyone is even encouraged to exercise, he or she must receive an appropriate physical exam.* This may be accomplished by in-house personnel or in conjunction with local hospitals or other health-care facilities.

A Corporate Fitness Center: Yes or No?

The decision to build an on-site fitness center depends to a very large degree on the size of the office or facility. Obviously, one would not expect to see a fitness center attached to local branch bank offices. Having an on-site center makes the most sense when the office or facility employs many people and alternative public fitness facilities are not readily available to employees.

Although a corporate fitness center can provide an excellent place for people to exercise under supervised conditions, such centers may not fill the entire need for exercise and may have some drawbacks. For example, unless the center is open to family members and for extended hours (possibly including weekends), its use may be limited. In order to facilitate use of the fitness centers, some companies have extended employee lunch hours. Others have introduced flexible lunch hours as well as flex-time.

At ICI Americas (see Section II for a description of their program), an employee who has an identified medical risk factor(s) may use the facility (with permission of his or her immediate supervisor) during midday or morning hours in addition to lunch and before and after work.

In almost every instance, the fitness centers we visited offer advantages to participants which would be difficult to duplicate elsewhere. The most important advantages are the availability of trained staff and quality programs, excellent procedures for charting and tracking exercise, and readily available exercise clothing (including on-site laundry services, towels, and hygienic supplies).

Many centers have exercise equipment that provides immediate feedback of the caloric equivalent of exercise. Many also have computerized record-keeping systems which employees can use to monitor their physical activity. These provide an incentive to exercise regularly.

Some facilities offer exercise classes in aerobics, low-impact aerobics, toning, jazzercize, stretching, and pre- and post-natal fitness. Special exercise programs designed to appeal especially to women, such as those for toning hips and thighs, also may be available.

Some fitness centers are closely linked to the company's medical department and may offer rehabilitation programs. For example, a whirlpool available at work may be used by someone recovering from an orthopedic problem. Without the facility at work, the person might not be able to return to the job as soon as would otherwise be possible.

Other Approaches to Fitness and Exercise

Many companies are either too small to have a fitness center or do not choose to have a fitness center. For example, at Ford Motor Company (see Section II for a description of their program),

> exercise education activities are delivered through three different options: exercise information, exercise education by demonstration, and exercise classes. Neither the UAW-Ford EAP or Total Health provides for the development of on-site exercise facilities or membership in health clubs. The purpose of exercise education is to encourage exercise through increased awareness and education, but not to provide unlimited continuing support of individual exercise programs.

Other companies providing fitness centers also want to encourage alternative exercise programs for their employees. As a case in point, Eastman Kodak emphasizes intramural sports and has 120 basketball teams, 130 volleyball teams, 220 softball teams, and 50 soccer teams.

Companies we contacted indicated that they supported or sponsored the following sports, many of which are organized by employees: hiking, racquetball, cross-country skiing, kayaking, jogging, tennis, pool, table tennis, basketball, volleyball, basketball, soccer, wallyball, softball, tennis, sailing, horseback riding, skiing, bowling, running, tennis, golf, and squash. Some companies also sponsored ballroom dancing and yoga.

At Holiday Corporation (see Section II for a description of their program), recreational programs are utilized extensively.

> The first step beyond the walls of the facility was into recreational sports such as volleyball, wallyball, racquetball, golf tournaments, a running team and tennis leagues. A strong recreational component has been helpful in attracting a variety of people who like to combine activity with competition and with social interaction. Recreation programs also provide an excellent method for people from various departments and levels within the company to meet and mix in a non-traditional business forum.

K-Tron Soder, Switzerland, contributed to a chalet for use by its employees and families for ski trips. Some companies provide outdoor bikes for employees to use while at work and have outside walking and jogging paths. Other companies provide video-cassette libraries with exercise tapes for employees to use at home. Many companies offer exercise seminars to encourage employees to exercise. Obviously, we find many approaches to encouraging fitness and exercise. In order to provide you with an example of an extensive fitness/wellness program, a detailed description of Burroughs Wellcome Co.'s program, specially prepared for this book, is included as Appendix A to this chapter. In addition, descriptions of programs provided by more than 50 other companies are included in Section II of this book.

Provider Services

Several major companies with their own fitness/wellness programs, including Johnson & Johnson and Control Data, serve as commercial providers for other companies. Other companies, such as Fitness Systems Provider Program, Medifit, and Fitness Development, Inc., specialize in helping companies, schools, and service organizations start and operate fitness programs. Descriptions of Fitness Systems' Provider Program and Fitness Development Inc.'s Provider Program, especially prepared for this book, are included as Appendixes B and C to this chapter.

Wellness Councils of America

For smaller companies, the Wellness Councils of America (WELCOA) that are developing across the United States may offer excellent guidance and support. William M. Kizer[2] provides the following description of WELCOA:

> Councils promote worksite programs and bring employers together with community health care providers and other resources already in existence. In that sense, there is a good symbiotic relationship between the councils and the community service providers (such as American Cancer society, YMCAs, and other nonprofit health organizations) and vendors (such as health clubs, hospitals, and stores that sell exercise equipment). Ideally, the professional staff

of the Wellness Council helps an employer devise an appropriate program—determine what is needed, like a stress management program—and then the council links the employer with a local provider.

The Wellness Councils serve a particularly important role in reaching the thousands of smaller companies that otherwise might be left behind in the fitness/wellness revolution.

WHAT'S AHEAD?

In Chapter 6 we provide a procedure for assessing the quality of and management commitment to fitness/wellness programs. We look at five important areas: (1) visible top management support, (2) strong and effective leadership, (3) excellence in medical testing, (4) convenient, easily accessible programs, and (5) comprehensive, diversified (and fun) programs.

APPENDIX A

BURROUGHS WELLCOME FITNESS PROGRAM

BURROUGHS WELLCOME CO.: WHO WE ARE

Burroughs Wellcome Co. is a research-based pharmaceutical firm head-quartered in Research Triangle Park, N.C. We are committed to the discovery and development of important medicines that offer significant benefit to mankind. Our 3,800 employees are engaged in biomedical research, the discovery and development of new medicines and the manufacture and marketing of pharmaceutical products.

Burroughs Wellcome Co. is the headquarters of the U.S. subsidiary of The Wellcome Foundation Limited, London. Wellcome is an international enterprise with companies in 50 countries and more than 18,500 employees worldwide. Here in the U.S. about 1,630 employees work at the Company headquarters and research laboratories in Research Triangle Park, about 1,570 work in the manufacturing facility in Greenville, N.C., and another 670 Sales Representatives are based around the country.

The Wellcome Foundation has a long tradition of outstanding biomedical research and boasts two Nobel Laureates among its scientists. Our consumer products include the cold medications ACTIFED® and SUDAFED® and the topical antibiotic NEOSPORIN.® Our prescription products include LANOXIN® for heart disease and SEPTRA®, a broad spectrum antibiotic. In the 1980s Burroughs Wellcome Co. introduced ZOVIRAX® the first drug to treat genital herpes, and the first drug to treat AIDS, RETROVIR®.

WELLCOME HEALTH: A WELLNESS PHILOSOPHY

Because health is our business, Burroughs Wellcome Co. has always felt a special commitment to the good health of its employees.

"We believe in creating an environment that brings out the very best in people," says Burroughs Wellcome Co. President Ted Haigler. "People have to feel good about themselves before they can feel good about their work, and that requires physical fitness and healthy lifestyles. We established Wellcome Health to help our employees achieve both."

Wellcome Health is a comprehensive wellness program available to all employees that reaches all aspects of corporate life. From the aerobics classes in the onsite fitness center to the menu in the Company cafeteria, Wellcome Health offers something for everyone.

Today's Wellcome Health program evolved from a long-standing philosophy about quality of life in the workplace. According to the Company's strategy statement, attracting and keeping the best people in the industry is a major goal. CEO Ted Haigler explains how Wellcome Health is part of that strategy.

"People are our most important resource, and how they feel about their work affects everything we do. Morale is the single most important factor in Burroughs Wellcome's success. It's a cliché, but in our case it's true that B.W. Co. is a family—employees, their spouses and children, everyone. Our goal is to keep that family spirit high.

"When you succeed at that, you can feel it everywhere—people sense they belong and are cared about. Recent attitude studies show that we're doing very well in this regard. Most employees feel good about Burroughs Wellcome. They see the Company's commitment to them in concrete things like benefits, Wellcome Health programs and the fitness center."

Before Wellcome Health took shape, the Company worked hard to create pleasant surroundings for employees. The architecture strives to provide attractive, relaxing space and light. Paintings and sculptures decorate the building. Landscaping offers patios, flower gardens and a reflecting pool. Jogging trails, Company sports and an annual Company run became part of a corporate lifestyle eager to grow into a formal wellness program.

HOW WE GOT STARTED

Although the literature claims corporate wellness programs have important economic benefits through reduced health care costs and decreased absenteeism, these were not the primary reasons for Wellcome Health.

"Those are valid goals, and wellness programs may achieve them. But our purpose in developing Wellcome Health was to enhance life in the workplace," says Betty Rowbotham, R.N., B.S., Wellcome Health program manager. "We wanted to create a climate of healthy lifestyles that would promote a sense of well being for employees and their families."

Rowbotham was hired in 1984 by the new director of Occupational Health and Safety, Lowrie Beacham, Ph.D. At that time the Company was expanding. A building adjacent to the site was being remodeled to include a fully-equipped fitness center and tennis courts. Employees had long been offered courses in stress management and presentations on health topics. Evening aerobics classes were held in the cafeteria. Dr. Beacham wanted a wellness program to tie all the pieces together and grow with the new facilities.

"We didn't argue for our program with statistics on reduced health care costs or absenteeism," Rowbotham says. "Even after four years, we find these outcomes very difficult to measure. We have six different medical benefits plans, for example, and it's very hard to monitor use. Absenteeism can be caused by so many factors other than health that we don't even try to correlate reduced absenteeism with fitness center use.

"To begin, we faced two problems: we had very little money for the program, and we didn't know how interested employees would be. Before we could ask management for a financial commitment, we had to demonstrate interest and effectiveness. So we started with a pilot project we called 'Be a Winner.' "

TWO KEY PROGRAMS ANCHOR
WELLCOME HEALTH

"Be a Winner" remains one of the two key programs in Wellcome Health. It began with 100 employees, 50 at Greenville and 50 at Research Triangle Park (RTP), who signed on to "meet the challenge" of improving their cardiovascular health on five measures: muscular strength, flexibility, endurance, percent of body fat and submaximal cardiovascular stress test. After evaluation, each received an exercise program, and they set as a goal to meet their exercise "prescriptions" for 12 weeks.

"We evaluated them again and found major improvements," Rowbotham says. "Ninety-two percent completed the program—and that was remarkable compared to the 30 percent average we found in the literature. So we took our results to management. They agreed that employees were interested and that the program could improve employee health. On those two bases we got the support we needed."

As 100 more employees signed on, Rowbotham turned her attention to a less structured three-month maintenance program designed to keep employees exercising after they completed "Be a Winner."

"We learned that monitoring was the key to employees' motivation." Rowbotham credits much of Wellcome Health's success to the intense involvement and enthusiasm of its two full and four part-time fitness instructors. Their interest and support have resulted in wide employee participation.

The second key to Wellcome Health's success is the Lifestyle Appraisal Questionnaire. "We recognized that a comprehensive wellness program had to be linked to physical evaluations and sound health counseling. The Lifestyle Appraisal is our link to the Burroughs Wellcome Health Center," Rowbotham says.

The Health Center asks all employees to fill out this detailed questionnaire on health habits and lifestyle. Results are used to offer individual counseling. Then employees are referred to Wellcome Health where they are given the opportunity to participate in group programs aimed at reducing their health risks.

Feedback from employees keeps Wellcome Health on track. Employees evaluate every program in which they participate. Questionnaires ask what they liked about the program, what they learned and what they still need. This year Rowbotham will hold several employee focus groups to get candid reactions to Wellcome Health and learn how it can better meet their needs. To keep information flowing, a bi-monthly Wellcome

Health newsletter is distributed at RTP and Greenville and is mailed to Sales Representatives. A Wellness Council is being set up to encourage employee participation in planning as Wellcome Health continues to evolve.

From "Be a Winner" and the Lifestyle Appraisal Questionnaire, Wellcome Health has grown to include targeted programs to reduce health risks such as smoking, high blood pressure and high cholesterol levels. These and Wellcome Health's wide selection of health education and information programs are outlined below.

THE WELLCOME HEALTH PROGRAM

Wellcome Health focuses on four health areas identified as major employee health risks—cardiovascular disease risk factors, smoking, obesity, and injuries resulting from car accidents. Employees are encouraged to reduce these risks by participating in Company programs in three general areas: physical fitness, health services and health education.

Fitness Center

Our 5,000 sq. ft. fitness center opened in 1986 at Research Triangle Park. The gym offers Keiser Strength Training equipment, exercise bicycles, ski and rowing machines and treadmills. Facilities include lockers, showers, changing rooms and separate space for aerobics and other classes. About 14 percent of employees use the center weekly. In 1987, a similarly equipped, 4,000 sq. ft. fitness center opened in Greenville.

Tennis Courts and Jogging Paths

Company grounds offer jogging paths through our beautiful 235-acre wooded site. Walking and jogging are major lunch-activities. The tennis courts are busy throughout the week.

"Be a Winner"

This fitness program challenges employees to meet specific exercise goals to improve cardiovascular health, muscle tone and endurance. The initial 12-week program evaluates employees on five measures of cardiovascular health, then prescribes an exercise regimen. Employees are monitored weekly as they turn in report sheets. The exercise physiologist charts their progress and offers support. More than 1,000 employees have taken the course; 80 percent still exercise regularly.

Aerobics Classes

Twelve-week classes are taught by 17 full and part-time instructors at the RTP and Greenville sites. Courses offer Early Bird Aerobics at 7:00 A.M.; Jazzercise, low impact, stretch and flex, high intensity/low impact, and Last Chance Aerobics at 5:30 P.M.; and karate. This is the only onsite Wellcome Health program for which a charge is made. The fee helps support instructors and serves as an incentive to keep employees coming to class.

Fitness Incentives

Incentives are designed to create long-term interest in fitness. The Company offers "flex lunch hours" to help employees schedule exercise. In another incentive plan employees earn "Well Bucks" by completing exercise programs, attending health education seminars, referring others to the program and competing in the Company run. They use them to purchase prizes. About 35 percent of employees participate.

Fitness Reimbursements

About 650 Sales Representatives are based around the country. This program reimburses them for 50 percent (up to $125) of the cost of an annual fitness club membership. Other services for this employee group include health education materials, referrals to stop smoking clinics and phone consultation on personal health and fitness.

Recreation

The Company-sponsored Unicorn Club offers athletic events including basketball, volleyball, softball, tennis, sailing, horseback riding, skiing and bowling. Activities are organized by employees and supported by Company funds.

Cafeteria Programs

To meet Wellcome Health goals for better nutrition, the Company cafeteria offers low-calorie and heart-healthy foods and posts caloric and sodium information on food selections.

HEALTH SERVICES

Lifestyle Appraisal

All employees are asked to complete a detailed lifestyle/health risk questionnaire. More than 96 percent of our work force has received this annual health risk assessment, which is a key aspect of the Wellcome Health program. The Health Center uses questionnaire results to offer individual counseling. Then employees are referred to Wellcome Health programs where they can participate to reduce their health risks. The Lifestyle Appraisal is supplied by the Center for Disease Control.

Physicals

All employees receive pre-employment and periodic physicals, including complete blood screens, cholesterol and HDL/LDL ratios, vision and audiometric exams and consultation with our contract physician.

CPR Training

Training and recertification are offered twice each year. Emergency Medical Response Teams of employee volunteers are trained and equipped with beepers to respond to medical emergencies at the work site.

Employee Assistance Program

EAP offers confidential counseling without charge to all employees and their families through an outside contractor. If a referral is made for emotional or crisis intervention, the Company pays for the first 10 visits and 50 percent of subsequent visits. EAP serves about 500 Burroughs Wellcome clients annually.

HEALTH EDUCATION

Health Month Programs

Health education programs are offered in conjunction with a health calendar. For example, February 1988 was American Heart Month. February programs focused on reducing cholesterol, increasing exercise, etc. Tables set up outside the cafeteria offered a one-minute "Save Your Sweetheart" quiz to test knowledge on cardiovascular health and offered a "Healthy Eater" prize of free lunches. Similar promotions appear for

National Nutrition Month in March, Cancer Control Month in April and so on throughout the year. These programs emphasize variety, since no one approach to weight loss or exercise will work for everyone.

Personal Health Counseling

The Wellcome Health coordinator helps employees design individual programs to reduce health risks.

Back Care

A survey assessed employee back care needs and a targeted program was developed. It includes screening through the Health Center, a 3-week education program and a 12-week exercise program for employees at high risk.

Cholesterol Awareness

Three-month training programs are supported by ongoing promotions through pamphlets and flyers. The course, called "How to Eat Low Fat in a High Fat World" is offered regularly.

Weight Management

Two 12-week weight-loss programs include individual counseling, nutrition programs, behavior modification programs and a weight-loss competition for employees. About 300 employees have participated at RTP.

Cancer Screening

Half-hour lunch programs on cancer screening and awareness train employees in breast self-exam, testicular self-exam and colorectal cancer.

Stop Smoking Clinics

These are held twice each year; about 100 employees attend annually. Clinics are supplemented by individual counseling and self-help training.

Blood Pressure Monitoring

The Company has installed two stations where employees can monitor their own blood pressure. This year, these stations were used 13,200 times.

Stress Management

Day-long programs offer training for a variety of specific stress situations, including family, career, personal maintenance, time management and assertiveness.

Seat Belt Safety

Literature and awareness programs encourage seat belt use among employees.

WELLCOME HEALTH RESULTS

Evaluations of Wellcome Health programs have come from Lifestyle Appraisal questionnaires of 1,310 employees surveyed in March of 1986 and 1987. That year the number of employees with high blood pressure fell from 9 percent to 6.8 percent; smoking declined from 17.6 percent to 15.9 percent; and failure to use seat belts was reduced from 30.6 percent to 16.8 percent.

Evaluations of cardiovascular health come from the "Be a Winner" program. Results of fitness measurements for 247 employees, after completing one full year with the program, include:

	Percent Change in Females	Percent Change in Males
Maximum VO$_2$ (efficient utilization of oxygen to heart and muscles)	27.1	24.9
Met level (level of cardiovascular improvement)	25.4	24.4
Upper body strength	109.0	61.2
Abdominal endurance	25.0	14.7
Percent body fat	-2.9	-8.2

"Thanks to our programs for cardiovascular health, we estimate that there are one million fewer heart beats at Burroughs Wellcome Co. every day," Rowbotham says. "Programs to reduce obesity resulted in total weight loss of more than one ton among our employees! We're succeeding—and maybe the best measure is that about 80 percent of our people now exercise regularly."

Rowbotham also reports that there is strong support from management. Benefits Director Kenn Kidd says Wellcome Health enhances the Company's benefits package. Though it's harder to measure, Rowbotham feels that employees' subjective responses are the most important measure of success.

"Employees tell us how much better they feel, how much more energy they have, " Rowbotham says. "One employee said she likes herself better since she's lost weight. Another told us how important exercise at the fitness center is to her because it is her private time to do something good for herself. That's the kind of impact we want to have on employees' lives."

APPENDIX B

FITNESS SYSTEMS

Fitness Systems has been designing, implementing and managing successful fitness programs for businesses since 1975. During that time, it has become the preeminent provider of corporate health and fitness services.

Fitness Systems has met the high standards of hundreds of companies nationwide. Our clients include companies in the fields of aerospace and defense, banking, petroleum, chemicals, electronics, food products, publishing, communications, consumer products and financial services.

In addition to its Los Angeles headquarters, Fitness Systems also maintains regional offices around the country. Within each region, the company employs degreed health and fitness professionals who implement, administer and supervise employee health and fitness programs.

As with individuals, it is easy for a company to start a fitness program. The challenge is to achieve long-term success, so that the full benefits are realized. Fitness Systems has the experience and proven track record to meet this challenge.

THE NECESSARY INGREDIENTS FOR A SUCCESSFUL FITNESS PROGRAM

For a company fitness program to be cost-effective, it must attract active participation well beyond the 10 to 15 percent of employees who are already exercising on their own initiative. It takes a thoughtfully planned program to motivate sedentary individuals to alter their lifestyles and start exercising regularly. But it is by activating this group that the company realizes the benefits and the program becomes cost-effective. These key ingredients are required to achieve this success.

Top Management Support

The success of any program starts at the top. Senior management must lead the way by actively participating and promoting the program to maintain a high rate of participation. Health and well-being are then perceived to be a vital part of the corporate culture.

Supervision

Professional supervision is another key element in a successful program. Well-qualified, enthusiastic fitness professionals can make the difference between shaping up and giving up. Personal interaction, ongoing program promotion, incentives, special events, sports training and a myriad of other factors all combine to achieve long-term success.

Facility

The exercise facility also plays an important role. It has to be carefully planned to assume peak-hour bunching is not stymied by bottle-necks. Bigger is not necessarily better, but well-balanced is. For every company there is a unique facility design which best achieves program goals on a cost-effective basis. Fitness Systems integrates these three ingredients to help plan and implement the best health and fitness program to meet the company's needs. Our primary services are described below.

OUR PRINCIPAL SERVICES

Fitness Systems specializes in safe, cost-effective fitness programs designed to meet the widely differing needs of corporate America. We provide the following consulting and management services.

Feasibility Studies

A successful fitness program begins with careful analysis. What does the company want to achieve with its program? What are the characteristics of its employee population? How large should the facility be? What type of fitness equipment is appropriate? How much does it cost to construct and operate a fitness facility? What is the potential payback?

Top management rightfully expects cogent answers to such questions before granting the authority to proceed. Our experienced consultants can answer all the key questions. A cost-benefit analysis, which helps to ensure that the potential value of the program far exceeds its cost, is included in every study we do. After on-site interviews and information gathering, we produce a comprehensive, written report which enables companies to make sound decisions. Such a formal report addresses the interests and possible concerns of top management and can be instrumental in consolidating their support for the program.

Facility Planning

If a company decides to establish a program and build a fitness center, Fitness Systems can consult on the design of the facility. Building on our earlier feasibility study, we work with architects and engineers to develop a suitable floor plan and the proper mix of equipment. Installations can range from a relatively inexpensive mini-facility to a completely equipped fitness center. At this stage, we also provide guidance on the myriad of items which tend to be overlooked, such as storage, aerobic dance flooring, track banking, emergency response system, sound system and computer specifications. In short, we will work with architects and engineers to ensure the facility contains the components needed to serve employees effectively and that it is laid out to facilitate convenient and safe exercise.

Turn-key Program Management

We have the tools and the experience to initiate and operate the fitness program for you. Our turn-key management service includes:

- Conducting a pre-program promotion to generate a higher level of interest.
- Setting guidelines for screening program participants.
- Providing well-qualified fitness professionals to supervise the facility.
- Prescribing individually tailored exercise programs.

- Encouraging ongoing participation through a variety of program promotion activities.
- Offering awareness seminars on topics such as nutrition, weight control and stress management.
- Evaluating the progress of individual participants.

In addition, quarterly reports are prepared for senior management on fitness program effectiveness, including participation rate and aggregate change in the group's fitness level. Thus, ongoing documentation is provided to justify ongoing support.

FITNESS SYSTEMS—PROVEN AND PROFESSIONAL

Fitness Systems has a proven track record at designing, implementing and managing employee fitness programs. We take great pride in that record and strive constantly to maintain our leadership position.

With our many years of experience, we know what it takes to make a program successful. We interact with top company management officials at all stages of program development; we work closely with the company's architects in finalizing facility plans; we coordinate with other program supporters to ensure smooth program implementation; and we make certain that every Fitness Systems employee has the knowledge, training and discipline to carry out his or her job in a professional manner.

APPENDIX C

FITNESS DEVELOPMENT, INC.

The Wellness Program for School District of Lancaster (PA) Staff

Meeting the needs of a diverse population within an educationally based workplace is the goal of the School District of Lancaster, PA. With over 18 sites and a total staff of 1,200 persons, the district began an ambitious program in February 1987. Fitness Development, Inc., a Lancaster-based health/fitness consulting firm, was hired to coordinate the program. Bill Sheely, president of Fitness Development, Inc., led the way in developing cooperation among the personnel committee, the school board, and the wellness steering committee. Sheely, who serves as a junior-high physical education teacher within the district, saw as an over-arching goal the need to curtail the rising cost of preventable health-care problems, as well as health-care problems directly related to stress and burnout.

After two full years of operation, the district has surveyed the staff and found that over 90 percent of the respondents observed an increase in wellness-based behaviors within their respective schools. Almost 90 percent stated that the wellness program has had a positive effect on their own personal health/lifestyle choices.

The program is designed annually around goals which are based on requests and suggestions from the staff and also on relevant issues pertaining to good health and wellness. Goals are communicated to each site by means of enthusiastic wellness facilitators and with the help of Mr. Raymond Menges, Director of Human Resources. Facilitators are vital since they serve as personal messengers for and to the steering committee and the president. They prepare information bulletin boards on such topics as nutrition, fitness, forthcoming events, and notes of interest. It is their caring that makes the program work!

The program's focus is not limited just to fitness, but rather looks at wellness from a total perspective, with emphasis on education and diversity. Some of the district's more successful projects are:

1. Fitness testing with computerized results and personalized feedback available in-house to all employees.
2. "Feelin' Fine" information newsletters written by President Sheely (over 80 percent of the survey respondents found these very helpful).
3. Blood-risk screening program at school sites utilizing a traveling hospital van (over 500 staff and family tested).
4. "Take-a-Hike," 20-minute stress-reduction walk program during school hours.
5. Wellness/health section developed for all libraries, including stress-reduction tapes and assorted books.
6. Special health education programs on such topics as diabetes, cancer, and cholesterol.
7. "Lose-a-Ton" weight-loss contest and other weight-loss programs, including the diet workshop program.

8. A variety of fitness offerings, including a volleyball league, basketball tourney, tennis tourney, exercise classes, and the availability of swimming pool and weight room at the high school.
9. Awards for miles-of-activity performed (aerobic-based).
10. Financial credit offered for amount of time spent within or outside of district on education and appropriate experiences related to health improvement.
11. A "wellness hotline" that directs calls from any staff member to Sheely's home office. The hotline is a particularly effective way to keep in touch with a large number of people and to assure a caring attitude. The phone is answered promptly and all calls are treated in strict confidence. This is a real wellness booster.

Effective January 1, 1989, a major goal of the district was to eliminate the use of all tobacco products within any district property. The district wellness program works closely with the American Lung Association to offer smoking cessation programs. In April 1989 the program received a Pennsylvania 2000 Award from the Interagency Council for Health.

ENDNOTES

1. Bernie S. Siegel, M.D., *Love, Medicine, and Miracles* (New York: Harper & Row, 1986), p. 66.
2. William M. Kizer, *The Healthy Workplace* (New York: John Wiley & Sons, 1987), p. 99.

CHAPTER 6

ASSESSING CORPORATE FITNESS/WELLNESS PROGRAMS[1]

The health of the people is really the
foundation upon which all their
happiness and all their powers as a
state depend.
Benjamin Disraeli

Corporate fitness/wellness programs differ from company to company, depending in large part on the size of the company and the size of the plant or office at a particular location. For smaller companies, as noted in Chapter 5, building and staffing a fitness center may not be a cost-effective or efficient way to deliver a quality program to employees.

Regardless of the method of delivery, the President's Council on Physical Fitness & Sports has suggested the following 12 criteria for effective employee fitness programs:

1. High-level Support.
2. Strong and Effective Leadership.
3. Availability.
4. Assessment and Periodic Testing.
5. Recording of Participant Progress.
6. Professional Environment.
7. Personalized and Effective Programs.
8. Total Programming.
9. Program Diversity.
10. Motivation and Incentives.

11. Effective Public Relations.
12. Enjoyable Programs.

Within these broad guidelines, fitness experts generally agree on five primary measures which may be used to assess the quality of fitness/wellness programs. These are important to you. Not only will they provide a way to measure a company's commitment to fitness, but they also will help you to assess the degree of commitment that a company has to its employees' overall quality of life and personal growth. These five measures are (1) visible top management support, (2) strong and effective leadership, (3) excellent medical testing programs, (4) convenient, easily accessible programs, and (5) comprehensive, diversified, and "fun" programs. Each is described below.

VISIBLE TOP MANAGEMENT SUPPORT

A born leader sees which way the
crowd is going and steps in ahead.

Visible top management support is essential to any successful fitness/wellness program. This support can be measured in three ways.

Management Commitment to the Programs

When assessing a program, you want to know if healthful practices (eating properly, exercising right, not smoking) are an accepted part of the corporate culture.

L. L. Bean (see Section II for a description of their program) provides an excellent statement which goes to the heart of commitment:

> We cannot, in good faith, ask employees to stop smoking at home if they are being exposed, unprotected, to fumes or dust at work. We cannot expect them to wear seat belts or follow safety rules off the job if we do not strive to provide a healthy and safe environment on the job. Similarly, the offering of aerobic exercise and stretching

programs to office workers cannot be separated from the offering of safe and ergonomically designed work stations.

Consider the example provided by Hallmark Cards (see Section II for a description of their program):

Hallmark has emphasized healthy, nutritional foods since the company's cafeteria service began in 1924. To encourage employees to develop and maintain healthy eating habits, the headquarters cafeteria provides a daily selection of "light" menu items as well as typed menus that feature the number of calories contained with each food item. In addition, food measured by the ounce in the cafeteria deli offers frozen and fresh yogurt along with fresh fruit. Special events, such as Valentine's Day's "Be Good To Your Heart" lunch program, promote positive eating practices by offering low-sodium, low-cholesterol and low-fat menu choices.

Du Pont insists that its employees always use seat belts. This may seem inconsequential on the surface, but in reality it represents a clear indication that Du Pont does care about its employees. Similarly, Du Pont's cafeterias offer nutritionally balanced foods.

IBM's "A Plan For Life Program" (see Section II for a description of their program) clearly demonstrates its level of commitment.

All regular and retired employees and their spouses and dependent children aged 15–22 are eligible to participate in company-paid and sponsored courses such as exercise, weight management, cardiopulmonary resuscitation and defensive driving. In addition, individuals may enroll in similar qualified courses provided by community or commercial organizations on a tuition assistance basis.

Kellogg's "Feeling Gr-r-reat Program" (see Section II for a description of their program),

provides a confidential diagnostic and referral service to help resolve personal problems or concerns. Assessment, counseling and referral services are available to all employees, dependents, and retirees at no cost. Concerns commonly dealt with include: marital and family relationships, finances, substance abuse, dependent care, legal issues, and any other concerns that might impact on the individual's mental wellness.

Merchandising the Programs to the Employees

Are the fitness facilities, where applicable, easily accessible, or are they off in the corner where you have to stumble across them to find out if they exist? Does it appear that the facility exists primarily for the use of "exercise buffs, " or does it actually promote fitness for everyone? Are there posters describing activities and events? Does the employee newsletter include a section on fitness/wellness topics? These are primary signs of how the company promotes the various fitness/wellness programs to the employees. (Note that many companies do not have a fitness center but do offer comprehensive wellness programs. Check to see that these are clearly defined and well publicized.)

Northwestern National Life Insurance Company (see Section II for a description of their program) promotes its programs by providing company time for them. Northwestern gives employees 30 minutes in addition to their 45-minute lunch break to participate in wellness activities, subject to supervisor approval.

Management Participation in the Programs

If the senior managers are participating actively and overtly, you can be sure that the company is committed to the program. So, as you assess a company's commitment, it would be useful to question who in top management is actively involved in physical fitness and how frequently they exercise and use the corporate fitness facilities (if available).

Utilization of fitness facilities by everyone, staff and management, can be another real indication that management wants to break down the corporate barriers and improve communications.

Increasingly, companies are doing away with the executive gyms and are encouraging all employees to use common facilities. This tends to be threatening to some managers but can have a very positive effect on employee morale, enhance the sense of teamwork, improve communications, and help to implement human relations strategies. Sharing facilities can be an indication that everyone is pulling together. Look for companies whose managers are willing to share in common facilities and do so regularly. (While sharing facilities is important, it should be noted that the lockers/showers provided for women normally have individual changing cubicles. This is important, since everyone should be included in the programs and women who, for example, have had radical mastectomies may desire privacy.)

STRONG AND EFFECTIVE LEADERSHIP

> Leadership is the art of getting
> somebody else to do something you
> want done because he or she wants
> to do it.

If the company has on-site fitness facilities, adequate staffing requires approximately one fitness professional (such as an exercise physiologist) for every 200 to 250 participants. Generally, depending on the program, about one third to one half of the eligible employees will be participants. So, if one thousand employees are eligible, the company should have two to three fitness professionals, in addition to appropriate management and clerical support for the program. These professionals should be included in both the planning and operation of the center.

But good staffing is much more than ratios of professionals to participants. *Dynamic, qualified leadership is absolutely essential to a quality fitness/wellness program.* In Appendix B of this chapter, we have included the job description for a fitness/wellness program director, supplied by Fitness Systems of Los Angeles, California. Note the wide range of technical and interpersonal skills that are required for dynamic leadership in a fitness/wellness program.

As noted in Chapter 5, although quality on-site staff is important to the success of fitness programs, many companies also draw heavily on outside resources. Courses in specialized fields such as nutrition, stress management, and smoking cessation are frequently staffed by outside experts on a course-by-course basis. Companies may arrange for courses using local outside resources such as representatives from the American Heart Association.

EXCELLENT MEDICAL TESTING PROGRAMS

> Happiness lies first of all, in
> health.
> *William Curtis*

In Section III, Dr. Frankl describes the importance of having an appropriate physical examination prior to commencing an exercise program. He also establishes some important benchmarks for those examinations.

Consider Pfizer's (see Section II for a description of their program) medical screening, for example:

> The medical screening procedure prior to participating in the Health and Fitness Program is perhaps one of the program's most important assets. Medical history, cardiovascular risk factor profile, blood and urine analysis, resting cardiogram, pulmonary and respiratory function tests, and complete physical examination are completed by Pfizer's physicians (Board Certified Cardiologist). The Health and Fitness Staff then conducts an exercise stress test, nutritional assessment, percent body fat analysis, and a musculoskeletal assessment.

As a part of their physical examination in the "Taking Care Program," The Travelers Companies (see Section II for a description of their program), even provides for a posture evaluation.

In addition to the baseline physical examination, many companies are offering specialized medical testing and do-it-yourself medical testing. Some examples are included below.

Pacific Telesis (see Section II for a description of their program) has located automated machines for monitoring blood pressure throughout the company. Weight scales are located next to each blood pressure machine, and the company encourages employees to check their blood pressure regularly by distributing articles about blood pressure and heart disease.

Similarly, Eastman Kodak (see Section II for a description of their program) provides Self-Care Centers. A responsibility of the medical department, these are small unstaffed stations in high-traffic areas where employees can weigh themselves, check their blood pressure, and get aspirin or other over-the-counter drugs from a vending machine.

Bank of America (see Section II for a description of their program) deals with high blood pressure using a hypertension self-management kit.

The hypertension self-management program is available on the request of a manager and comes as a kit including information on the importance of the detection of hypertension, a digital blood pressure monitor, wall posters, a videocassette, and instructions on how to run the program. Employees who choose to participate, send in their blood pressure readings to the registered nurse in Corporate Health Programs who screens each form and replies by letter to each one. Employees with elevated readings are contacted by phone and offered support in ways to lower their pressure.

ARCO's (see Section II for a description of their program) LIFELINE program offers a unique approach to regular monitoring of employee health.

It provides an innovative approach that addresses personal welfare and longevity, as well as human performance. This is accomplished through a personal Health Risk Assessment, which enables the employee to take direct responsibility for his or her current health status. This voluntary program requires the employee, through an interactive computer program, to answer questions about personal habits and family health background. In addition, serum cholesterol is obtained at the same time. The employee then receives a personalized report that compares him or her with norms established in a broad industrial population.

IBM, through its "Voluntary Health Assessment" program (see Section II for a description of their program), generates a health profile for each employee based on age, lifestyle, heredity, and other pertinent personal information. It then identifies an individual's risk of developing a particular illness and suggests steps the person can take to significantly lower that risk.

Northwestern National Life Insurance Company (see Section II for a description of their program) provides an annual fitness assessment.

Each year, employees may participate at no cost in a fitness assessment conducted by the wellness director, a certified fitness specialist. It measures factors such as height and weight, body composition, blood pressure, cardiovascular endurance, muscular strength and flexibility. Participants receive a detailed description of their personal results and suggestions on ways to improve their overall level of fitness.

CONVENIENT, EASILY ACCESSIBLE PROGRAMS

Here's your hat,
what's your hurry?
Bartley C. Costello

One of the best predictors of a program's success is convenience to the participants. Convenience is measured both in terms of physical location and the time the facilities are open and available to the employees. Companies and employees benefit most when those employees who do not already exercise on their own are attracted to the company's program. Normally, 10 to 15 percent of a company's employees have an established interest in fitness and will exercise regularly, regardless of what programs the company may offer. To be successful, a fitness/wellness program must reach the remaining employees. *Convenience is essential.*

How do you measure convenience? Look at the hours the facilities are open and the hours employees may use them. For example, do you permit flexitime, and may employees exercise when they want to? As a practical matter, flexitime is not always possible, and especially if production lines are involved. In any event, the facilities should be open before and after working hours (usually two hours after the end of the workday) and during lunch periods. Some facilities are open on weekends. In more rural areas, families are often permitted to use the facilities. Sometimes their use is limited to non-peak hours.

Another measure of convenience is proximity to the facilities. For example, it may be more efficient for a company in a metropolitan area to offer employees memberships in a nearby health club or YMCA than to build a fitness facility. The health club is likely to be open longer hours and on weekends so that employees who live nearby can use the facility at their convenience. Many employees, however, do not have the time to use facilities on the weekends and are better served by coming to work early three times a week, or using on-site facilities during their lunch hours.

COMPREHENSIVE, DIVERSIFIED (AND FUN) PROGRAMS

> Most people want to be
> delivered from temptation, but
> would like to keep in touch.
> *Robert Orben*

Another primary measure of a quality fitness/wellness program is its diversity and comprehensiveness. Each individual's fitness program should be carefully designed to help him or her reach the goals set during the initial medical/fitness screening. Programs should be challenging, vigorous, noncompetitive, and follow the basic principles of exercise science.

Programs that offer satellite activities such as stress management and nutrition counseling and smoking cessation classes are particularly effective in helping employees maintain healthful lifestyles. Many companies find that fitness programs are more successful when spouses and families of employees are included. Also, offering special workshops in the evenings and on weekends can build employee interest and participation. Exercise becomes the catalyst for helping participants to achieve other goals they may have set for themselves, such as losing weight or improving in their chosen sport.

Group classes, in addition to individual activities, should be available for those who prefer the companionship and social aspects of a group environment. Jogging, swimming, or stationary bicycles should be available for those who prefer to exercise alone.

A quality program should offer the opportunity for such programs as nutritional guidance (and weight counseling), family counseling (including marital and child), stress counseling, cardiopulmonary resuscitation (CPR) classes, hypertension control, safety in the home and workplace, and referrals to EAPs. Many companies are offering programs dealing with low-back pain.

Some companies employ counselors with masters degrees in social work who specialize in counseling. These counselors provide active support and help to employees facing critical life problems. Such counseling may prevent illness and contributes to personal growth.

Finally, the program should be enjoyable. Fun, as well as

physical and psychological benefits, should be a major objective of the program. If you can't really enjoy yourself, you will likely drop out. This doesn't mean that the level of physical activity should be slackened. Rather, it means there must be variety, companionship, stimulation, and caring on the part of the fitness staff.

To give you an idea of what an extensive program looks like, we include the schedule for PepsiCo's Health and Fitness Program as Appendix A to this chapter. In addition, we are including as Appendix B the job description for a program director, provided by Fitness Systems.

WHAT'S AHEAD?

Earlier in the book we noted that the movement of Corporate America into fitness/wellness programs is well underway. As we interviewed executives, we found that many expressed ideas which likely will determine the future of these programs for years to come. These and other comments from senior managers are included in Chapter 7.

APPENDIX A

1989 PEPSICO HEALTH ENHANCEMENT PROGRAM OFFERINGS[2]

1989 PEPSICO HEALTH ENHANCEMENT PROGRAM OFFERINGS

I. Fitness Profile Testing—used to determine the individual's initial level of fitness; to aid in the development of an individualized exercise prescription; to provide a baseline of information from which we can then quantify the amount of progress achieved in the first 6 months and each year thereafter.

Test Administration
1. Body Composition
   a. Skinfold
   b. Girth
2. Muscular Endurance/Strength
   a. Handgrip
   b. Benchpress
3. Flexibility
4. Abdominal Endurance
5. Aerobic Assessment

II. Workout Series
   A. High Impact Aerobics
      1. Early Bird
      2. Exertone
      3. Powertone
      4. Exerflex

   B. Low Impact
      1. Beginner aerobics
      2. Exercise Plus
      3. Bottom Line

III. Physical Conditioning/Training Program*
   1. Yoga
   2. Oyama Karate
   3. Stretching
   4. Ski Conditioning

IV. Recreational/Intramural Activities
   1. Tennis
   2. Racquetball
   3. Squash
   4. Soccer
   5. Golf

---

*We have a video library on a variety of health promotion and disease prevention issues that employees may borrow at any time (i.e., breast cancer, preventing heart attack, back pain, childhood illnesses, etc.). High and low impact aerobic tapes are also available for employees to use when the aerobic class area is not in use.

    6. Swimming
    7. Volleyball
    8. Bowling

V. Health Styles Series
    1. Defensive driving
    2. Weight Watchers

VI. Brown Bag Seminars
    1. Beware of Cholesterol
    2. Work and Family: Combining Commitments
    3. Reprogramming Negative Self-Talk
    4. Nutrition and Disease Prevention
    5. Praise and Child Rearing
    6. "Back" Talk
    7. Stress Reduction Techniques for Today's Family
    8. Eat to Win
    9. Time Management Tips for Home and Work
    10. Power Eating
    11. Choices in Childbirth: Part 1, 2, and 3
    12. Stress Free Living
    13. New Parents Returning to Work
    14. Dining Out with Discretion
    15. Change Your Thinking; Change Your Life
    16. How to Talk to Your Child about S-E-X
    17. Humor to Serious Business
    18. Self-Esteem
    19. A Personal Safety Program—Protect Yourself
    20. Dress for Success
    21. Today's Father
    22. On the Job Relaxation Techniques
    23. Taking Charge of Change Skills for the 90s: Part 1—The Stressors; Part II—Taking Charge
    24. Protect Yourself

VII. Incentive Programs
    1. Fitness Frenzy
    2. 10,000 Sit-Ups Abdominal Club
    3. Turkey Trot

VIII. PepsiCo Sponsored Programs
Corporate Invitational Tennis Tournament (CITT)

IX. Health Fitness Newsletter
   Monthly health and fitness newsletter

X. Nutrition Analysis
   Five-day dietary recall analysis

APPENDIX B

JOB DESCRIPTION—PROGRAM DIRECTOR

JOB SUMMARY

The program director is ultimately responsible for overseeing all fitness center activities; supervises staff; ensures coordination of the development and implementation of fitness programs, health education activities, program promotion and special events; ensures proper maintenance of participant records; reports to Fitness Systems management and company liaison on program effectiveness; ensures maintenance of equipment and facility; ensures safe, clean environment of the center; carries out other projects and duties which contribute to program effectiveness as assigned by Fitness Systems and company management; reports to regional vice president or regional director.

JOB DUTIES AND RESPONSIBILITIES

Oversees all fitness center and health promotion activities: Ensures that participants' needs are met satisfactorily; verifies that fitness center activities comply with established Fitness Systems and company management standards; and coordinates daily, monthly and quarterly reporting activities.

Supervises staff: Hires, trains, and discharges personnel, as necessary; delegates work assignments; approves staff schedules; evaluates staff performance and ensures staff development.

Coordinates the development, integration and implementation of fitness programs, health education activities, program promotion and special events; devises periodic programs to encourage facility use, stimulate interest in the program, and improve cardiorespiratory and muscle conditioning; creates graphic displays and other props as health education tools; prepares periodic newsletters to update participants on fitness center programs; plans and oversees special health and fitness events (e.g., health fair, corporate races, etc.).

Ensures proper maintenance of participant records: Maintains records of participants' (1) attendance at fitness facility, (2) exercise frequency, (3) changes in physiological conditioning, (4) injury or illness incidents at the facility, and (5) membership payroll deductions or fee payments. Retests participants and updates exercise program; ensures follow-up with participants with low facility attendance; oversees all computer operations; and verifies records for accuracy.

Interfaces with company management and peripheral departments. Maintains ongoing communication with Fitness Systems, company management, medical department and other function areas, as appropriate; prepares annual fitness center budget; develops annual operating plan for the facility; handles inquiries by media and other interested parties; refers callers, when applicable, to appropriate Fitness Systems official or to the company management.

Conducts fitness testing: Evaluates cardiorespiratory and muscle conditioning of program participants; prescribes exercise program; and instructs participants on proper techniques for carrying out recommended exercise program.

Ensures safe and clean environment at the center: Oversees maintenance and janitorial contracts; ensures equipment is well-maintained and operating properly.

Reports to Fitness Systems management and company liaisons on program effectiveness: Ensures timely production of management reports for submittal to company contacts and Fitness Systems.

JOB REQUIREMENTS

Graduate degree in physical education, exercise physiology, kinesiology or health education from an accredited college or university; prior experience in program management and staff supervision; certificate in cardiorespiratory pulmonary resuscitation and first aid certifications mandatory; communication skills to instruct and interact effectively in a corporate setting also required.

ENDNOTES

1. The authors gratefully acknowledge the input of William Horton, President, Fitness Systems, Los Angeles, CA, in the preparation of this chapter.
2. Provided by Frank J. LoCastro, Ed.D, Manager, Corporate Fitness, PepsiCo, Inc. Used with permission.

CHAPTER 7

THE FUTURE OF FITNESS/WELLNESS PROGRAMS

There is no special limit on the
pursuit of excellence.

The emergence of fitness/wellness programs and their rapid
growth during the past few years is indicative of the evolutionary
nature of this movement. Based on our research and interviews,
we anticipate accelerating growth of these programs. Moreover,
we anticipate an integration of these programs into the general
rubric of existing organizational behavior models.

At present, some fitness/wellness programs are tangential to
the central focus of organizational development. As they continue
to gain heightened visibility, however, we can expect them to become an integral part of a broad organizational development
model that includes all those services and programs that help employees cope more effectively with a rapidly changing business environment. Later in this chapter we will share some viewpoints of
managers we interviewed who clearly see the need to expand
management's conceptualization of what we broadly call "human
services," of which the fitness/wellness movement is a vital, growing part.

As we noted earlier in the book, the fitness/wellness movement speaks to changes in management attitudes and therefore to
changes in managers' attitudes. The acceptance of the principles
of caring management by managers, and the integration of those
principles into their management styles, is likely to be the single
most significant challenge to face Corporate America during the
next 10 years.

In this chapter we will examine three topics:

1. *The changing philosophy toward fitness/wellness programs.*
2. *The integration of fitness/wellness programs into Corporate America.* Specifically, how these programs will intermesh with training, communications, and numerous other programs directed toward employee growth and development.
3. *The challenges presented to management and the changing of managerial attitudes.* Specifically, management's adaptation to the more humanistic, caring work environment presently emerging and likely to continue in most companies for the next 10 years.

THE CHANGING PHILOSOPHY TOWARD WELLNESS AND ILLNESS

Minds are like parachutes: they
only function when open.

Despite the widespread interest in fitness today, many companies still reward illness and provide little recognition for wellness. It appears that our society still clings to old, neurotic behavior patterns that not only encourage ill health by rewarding it, but also largely ignore the healthy individual who contributes much more to the organization than his or her unhealthy counterpart. Sick people are rewarded with time off from work and the payment of their medical bills. In addition, they become the subject of at least moderate attention from co-workers and supervisors. To some degree, being sick places one in a position of enjoying special recognition.

This "culture of sickness" begins when a child is in school. The only socially acceptable way to get some time off from school is to be sick. Also, an illness may provide the opportunity to receive some extra caring from parents, relatives, and friends.

In addition to rewarding the sick, many companies still do not provide healthy corporate environments and "healthy" examples for their employees. *Healthy environments and good examples of wellness are absolutely critical to establishing good health as an integral part of the corporate way of life.*

Rewarding the Well

If wellness programs are to be successful, good health must be rewarded and sickness discouraged. During our research and discussions with managers, we heard many excellent ideas which can be implemented to encourage healthy lifestyles and wellness among employees. Several are listed below:

1. Permit employees to accumulate sick leave days and pay the employee for half of these days when he or she retires or otherwise terminates employment.

2. At the end of each year, convert each unused sick day to one-half day of additional vacation for the following year, or pay the employee a "health bonus" equivalent to one half of that year's unused sick days.

3. Establish "perfect attendance" recognition programs. Award perfect attendance publicly.

4. Provide each employee with a record of his or her medical insurance costs (including costs incurred by dependents) for the year, along with the average medical expenses per company employee. If the employee had lower insurance costs than the average, credit the difference toward his or her medical insurance deductible for the following year.

5. Provide reduced medical insurance deductibles and co-payments for those who maintain weight within prescribed ranges, maintain cholesterol within appropriate levels, use seat belts regularly, exercise regularly, and don't smoke.

6. Provide regular and extended physical exams and complete health-risk assessments for all employees, including exercise cardiograms. Based on the results, recommend appropriate physical exercise and behavior modification programs (such as smoking cessation or weight loss).

7. Consider extending the physical examination and health-risk appraisal programs described in item six, above, to dependent family members, keeping in mind that roughly two thirds of medical insurance costs are for dependents. Also, note

that a major cause of parent absenteeism from work is the need to care for sick children at home. This suggests the necessity of on-site child care centers that provide facilities and staff to care for children who are sick.

8. Reward individuals who make special contributions to the organization with additional vacation. This unique incentive might be used in place of or in conjunction with performance bonuses. It has an advantage over monetary bonuses, however, in that it provides time for relaxation and recuperation—which may lead to a reduction in stress and also may foster creativity.

Finally, we note that as the assimilation of minorities and immigrants into the work force accelerates, wellness programs will be in greater need because many of these people traditionally lack insurance coverage and, therefore, may have untreated health problems or may be suffering from poor nutrition. It will be especially important for companies to get these people to at least a basic level of health and wellness awareness and then start them on the road to following healthful practices.

Developing a "Good Health" Corporate Climate

Management must establish a healthy corporate culture if it wants employees to be healthy. To start, this means that top managers especially must set a healthy example by not smoking, keeping weight under control, and exercising regularly (and, where possible, doing so visibly).

In addition, the company must establish policies encouraging healthy practices, including not smoking, alcohol moderation, and seat belt use. Nonsmoking is essential. Also, the company should deemphasize the use of alcohol, especially at company meetings, cocktail parties, and other outings.

Similarly, the company must provide an atmosphere free of pollutants and minimize physical stress. This points toward ergonomics and a reexamination of office designs and space utilization.

The fundamental idea is to present the employee with a corporate culture emphasizing good health through exercise, recreation, good nutrition, not smoking, and not drinking, while at the same time setting the example for the corporate culture by visible actions on the part of management. Management must walk the way it talks—and especially so when it comes to good health habits, healthy working environment, and the rewarding of wellness.

THE FUTURE OF EMPLOYEE ASSISTANCE PROGRAMS

> If you want to be the picture of
> health, make sure you have a happy
> frame of mind.

Employee Assistance Programs (EAPs) are likely to become increasingly more important within the whole fitness/wellness framework. This will result largely from the diversity of EAP programs (see Chapter 5 for a listing) and the fact that many companies will be looking for programs to help employees deal with emotionally stressful situations. At present, however, only a limited number of these programs and services are available to most employees. The primary growth of EAPs will result from the delivery of more of the existing programs and services to additional employees rather than the addition of new programs to the list, which is already comprehensive.

As we suggested, *a primary area of growth will be in programs designed to reduce employee and manager stress and help employees and managers deal with stress more effectively.* Companies will try to help employees help themselves in crucial areas such as money management, for example. Money management is a primary cause of marital problems and a source of difficulty for many people. Money problems clearly cause stress. Similarly, on-site day care centers will increase, as will the availability of more flexible scheduling. These not only will reduce stress, but also will help in attracting employees—an important consideration in a tight labor market.

With respect to handling stress, more programs will be offered in those areas which are now viewed as somewhat "fringy" by both conservative managers and employees. These will include yoga, meditation, self-hypnosis, imaging, and similar programs. Again, the example set by upper-level managers will be critical to the successful implementation of these programs. Just as Greyhound's Chairman Teets climbs 19 flights of stairs to his office, other senior managers will have to break out of traditional molds and become actively involved with the more experimental techniques such as meditation or yoga.

Education is clearly the primary vehicle in developing an awareness of the advantages of being healthy and an understanding of how to be a well person. Education is also necessary to get the employee's attention. Education will emphasize accurate dissemination of information on ways to become healthy, as well as relating this information to each employee's individual health-risk profile. The individual must be educated to understand how lifestyle directly affects one's ability to cope with the working environment. Education will be a large part of the "hook" which will get people involved with becoming healthy.

Finally, *EAP programs and courses are likely to become more behavior-modification-oriented and less goal-oriented.* This means stressing a behavioral change such as adoption of new eating habits, for example, which, over time, will result in weight loss or reduction in cholesterol level, rather than suggesting a diet to accomplish the same goals. The emphasis increasingly will be on promoting life-long living patterns which stress good health and good health maintenance. For example, *we can expect to see more ongoing, individualized programs focused on teaching those managers who cause employee stress to be less stressful.*

The Financial Motive

The motive for EAPs will largely remain based on the bottom line with respect to reducing absenteeism and medical costs. An excellent example is provided in a June 24, 1988 *Wall Street Journal* article on corporate prenatal care plans.[1] The article noted that it cost AmeriTrust $1.4 million in benefits for the premature birth of a baby girl. Half of the medical costs paid by Sunbeam at Cowhatta, La., for a 530-employee plant was for the care of four premature babies. The article also notes that many companies have developed their own prenatal care programs, and more than 150 have adopted a prenatal health care program provided by the March of Dimes Birth Defects Foundation.

Similarly, more companies will offer back-injury avoidance programs. We can expect to see employees who lift and otherwise stress the back muscles to be instructed in back stretching and warm-up exercises and be given the time at work to perform those exercises.

THE FUTURE OF FITNESS PROGRAMS

> Do not follow where the path may
> lead. Go instead where there is no
> path and leave a trail.

Being physically fit is becoming a way of life for many people. The media focuses on those who are slim, trim, and in good physical condition. This change in attitude toward fitness may be best exemplified by comparing the movie stars of only 20 years ago (such as Marilyn Monroe) with today's Jane Fonda and Cher. Clearly, being fit and trim is now the culturally accepted norm. *The cultural shift toward fitness will probably be the single most important factor in promoting fitness and exercise programs. Exercising, sweating, and keeping in shape are now culturally acceptable.*

The fitness movement faces three important hurdles in reaching its full potential:

1. Getting those people who don't already exercise regularly to become involved in exercise programs.
2. Providing the proper physical examinations to people before they start exercise programs.
3. Regularly monitoring those who exercise and motivating them to continue to exercise.

Motivating the Couch Potatoes

To some extent, the difficulty in getting those who do not exercise to start regular exercise programs will be mitigated by the increasing social pressure. As noted above, being "fit" is in and being fat is out. Beyond the social pressure however, employers will have a tough job selling some couch potatoes on exercise. Behavior modification takes time, and the individual must be convinced that it is in his or her best interest to exercise.

A fitness facility can provide motivation for some employees mainly because of its convenient access to a wide variety of exercise equipment, programs, and staff. The existence of a fitness center also makes a very positive statement about the company's attitude toward exercise and fitness. Finally, since many fitness centers increasingly will become rehabilitation centers in the future, injured workers will find the whirlpool and appropriate rehabilitation exercise equipment readily accessible. These people will be encouraged to continue exercise as a part of their ongoing rehabilitation programs.

Providing Proper Physical Examination

Obtaining a proper physical exam before commencing a regular exercise program is essential. Not to do so may be fatal! Some employers presently do not provide any physical exams for employees, let alone stress cardiograms. Yet, such physicals are absolutely essential to fitness programs because the results are the basis for establishing an appropriate, individualized exercise program for each employee. (See Dr. Frankl's comments on physical examinations in Section III.)

Many companies do not have the on-site medical staff (including board-certified cardiologists and orthopedic physicians) or the facilities and equipment needed to give an appropriate physical exam or set up an exercise program for each employee and, perhaps, family members as well. Providing these comprehensive physicals can be expensive; however, in the long run, they likely will produce very positive end results by helping in early disease detection and by establishing a solid base for exercise, weight reduction, and other individualized wellness programs.

In the future, physical exams, or the parts of the exam involving stress cardiograms, likely will be performed on a contract basis by local hospitals. The results will be provided to an exercise physiologist (as well as to the employee's physician) who will work individually with each employee to establish an exercise program with other appropriate wellness elements. Such an approach is already in operation at the Tucson (Arizona) Medical Center, where a medical staff of over 80 physicians of various specialties provide an office-based wellness program and a screening process for high-risk individuals.

Monitoring and Motivating Exercise Programs

The exercise physiologist will have to meet regularly with each employee and assist the employee in monitoring his or her progress. This type of monitoring already exists at many corporate fitness centers. It is unlikely, however, that more than five percent of the total work force will ever have access to a corporate fitness center. The work, therefore, of the exercise physiologist will be of a somewhat missionary nature.

Physiologists will travel from location to location, meeting individually and regularly with employees in exercise programs. The physiologist's work will be especially important for those who are not fit, those with high-risk factors, and those with orthopedic problems. Concurrently, the physiologist will meet with those who do not exercise and, based on the results of physical exams, suggest appropriate exercise programs.

The physiologist will be the key link in the motivating and monitoring process, helping individuals to stay on proper exercise programs through a combination of motivation and direction techniques. In addition, the physiologist will provide technical direction and oversee specific programs in areas such as back care.

Many people who have physically demanding jobs think they are in shape because they "exercise" at work. This is just not the case. These people will require the special attention of the exercise physiologist if they are to avoid injury and receive an appropriate exercise program.

INTEGRATION OF FITNESS/WELLNESS PROGRAMS INTO THE ORGANIZATIONAL STRUCTURE

> Don't be afraid to go out on
> a limb—that's where the
> fruit is.

At the present time, some fitness/wellness programs are tangential to the main thrust of most companies. Organizationally, they

generally fall within the scope of the vice president for human resources and may or may not be closely linked with the medical department. In some cases they are loosely linked with corporate
training programs. What will be the place of fitness/wellness programs in the future?

Within the context of developing a caring approach to employees, we asked managers what they felt would be their greatest
challenges during the next 10–15 years. They indicated several
important ones, listed below:

1. The need for managers to understand their employees.
2. The need to provide a stable working environment.
3. The need to stress performance management.
4. The need to provide a more horizontal integration of
   management.
5. The need to keep employees motivated.

The Need to Understand Employees

A number of the managers we interviewed spoke of the need for
all managers to develop a greater understanding of the sociologi-
cal changes in our society and the profound effects these changes
have had on employees over the past two or three decades. In addition, these managers also indicated that the effective manager
of tomorrow will have to have a deeper understanding of human
psychology.

Managers also noted that, for the past two generations, most
of our children have been experiencing relatively open environments where, in large part, they have been able to call the shots.
They go into school systems that cater to the individual. If they
are unhappy in school, they protest. They make demands and they
get attention. This leaves them with a set of experiences that leads
them to believe that they should have control over most, if not all,
aspects of their lives.

In addition, with the breakdown of the traditional family,
children increasingly have become accustomed to loose and
largely unstructured relationships. For example, children not infrequently have to share the same household with children from
other marriages.

Managers pointed out that integrating these younger employees into the work force, especially where a large organization is involved, is not a simple process. If these young employees came out of tightly bound nuclear families, the fit into a big corporation generally is much easier.

Corporate America needs people who identify with the organization. But managers are dealing with many people who don't find that "identification" a particularly attractive or operational value. Most of their prior affiliations have been very loose and changeable. Accommodating these values and behaviors into the corporate environment can be a real management challenge, requiring a deep understanding of motivational and team-building techniques.

Organizations demand subordination of the individual to the organization. The Japanese have learned this fact. With so many people crammed into a small space, their whole lifestyle and culture is built around the principle that the individual must be subordinate to the larger group. By contrast, our culture has been based on individualism and expansion. As the frontiers close, we will have to change. But in the interim, managers must recognize that our culture is not conducive to the development of individuals who are easily assimilated into large-scale organizations.

The Need to Provide a Stable Working Environment

Carl G. Sempier, past President of Mannington Resilient Floors,[2] indicated that most employees are looking for work environments which are stable, secure, and provide challenges and rewards. He noted that this contrasts with advertisements showing the "beautiful people" taking risks and working in high-stress, volatile positions. He stressed the need for environments which allow the employee to become involved, environments that are open and receptive, not stifling, where a person can reach his or her potential and where there is opportunity to excel. That may sound rather idealistic, but we heard this theme repeated again and again.

Mr. Sempier stressed that employees want a work environment that will let them sleep at night and not lie awake worrying at 3 A.M. *All of this speaks to a physical, mental, and spiritual attitude.* He further noted that he believes employees will choose stability and security over higher wages.

The Need to Stress Performance Management

Mr. Sempier also noted that managers will need to stress performance management, using teams of people as well as recognition programs to try to break down the barriers that have arisen between employers and employees during the last 10 years. Performance evaluations will start to change as people are evaluated in a team setting rather than as sole contributors.

Bonuses and promotions will be predicated on the ability of individuals and managers to perform well as a part of a team. This means that senior managers will have to convince subordinates that they can be trusted to evaluate them on the basis of teamwork rather than on individual accomplishments. Concurrently, this will reduce the need for the individual "superstars," who frequently attain their stardom at the expense of others within the organization. Managers will have to learn to manage teams and to rate subordinates according to individual as well as teamwork measures.

The Need to Provide a More Horizontal Integration of Management

Mr. Sempier further noted that the most significant forthcoming change is toward horizontal integration of management. Vertical, pyramidal management involves sending messages up and down. Senior managers are forced to adjudicate between managers on the same level and deal with egos. Similarly, managers tend to find fault with their contemporaries and look for ways to shine, often at the expense of others. In the future, there must be horizontal integration, with rewards for achieving results as part of a team.

THE CHALLENGE OF KEEPING EMPLOYEES MOTIVATED

> As I grow older I pay less
> attention to what men say. I
> just watch what they do.
> *Andrew Carnegie*

Managers noted that one of the important challenges they face is to make the work interesting and exciting so that employees want to stay on the job. But mangers told us that they frequently took the easy way out, and found economic incentives easier to use. Managers should strive to make employees want to stay. Every day managers should motivate and challenge their employees and provide a good working environment so employees voluntarily will want to continue the relationship—not "shanghai them" by keeping them in deep water until it is management's pleasure to drop them off on the beach. The best relationships are built on voluntary interaction, not dependency.

How does management keep employees excited and challenged, especially when the opportunities for promotions are limited? William Noyes, Vice President, Human Resources, Hershey Foods,[3] indicated that they were forming more task groups to give participants more exciting things to do. Hershey is also placing more people on temporary assignments and making a lot of lateral transfers to provide opportunities for growth and exploration. Mr. Noyes noted:

> A large percentage of our employees work in rural areas, and we find that they typically are more productive than employees in metropolitan areas. They probably have a better work ethic. We have also learned through experience that our employees want to be treated as human beings. If we let them know what we need, relate this to their future, provide them with incentives, make them a part of the action, delegate more to them, and really give them a chance to participate—they will respond positively.
>
> Four or five years ago, we experimented with a new confectionery plant in Virginia and reduced the layers of management as well as the different categories of employees that we would normally have. In other locations, supervisors wore white hats and white shirts—

could have been looked upon as the "good guys," and we wanted to stress at this new location that everyone was important. We eliminated the different uniform colors, did away with special parking places for management, eliminated time clocks and placed everyone on salary, and attempted to create more of an atmosphere of "team work" by stressing similarities rather than differences. We also had all employees on basically the same benefit plans.

In addition, we reduced the different pay categories to as few as possible. We also trained a certain number of plant employees as replacements for the next level of positions above them, and paid them for that higher level function even though they would not be in that higher level job all the time. This paying for the higher level skill encouraged employees to upgrade their skills and be available when needed, and further encouraged the "team spirit."

Our overall experience from these changes was a more highly motivated group of employees, a need for fewer supervisors, and a reinforcement that we can all gain through increased productivity.

An interesting, but unexpected, experience resulting from all this really brings the message home. In other locations, our Medical Departments typically spend time with employees on disability and encourage them to come back to work as soon as they are deemed physically able. At this particular plant, we found our employees so highly motivated that they often attempted to come back to work before they were ready—and our Medical Department had to watch them to make sure they did not come back prematurely.

Mr. Spencer, National Director of Human Resources of Laventhol & Horwath,[4] noted that at his company,

We have high employee turnover. Retention is a real concern. Our goal is to keep more people for longer periods of time—especially the more productive people. We do this by some incentive compensation, performance appraisals, counseling, and recognition of accomplishments.

We need to provide more recognition. We thought that only marginal people wanted recognition. I think the higher performers want more of it and thrive on it. Compensation is score-keeping for many employees. We are experimenting with three kinds of compensation plans.

I think we make more profit and give better service by motivating enthusiastic employees who feel the organization is trying to do all it can to help them grow professionally and help them with their problems. I think you get productivity by training, motivating, and by showing concern.

Raymond M. Fino, Vice President, Human Resources, Warner-Lambert,[5] indicated that they were increasing challenges by:

> stressing job rotation from line to staff, between operational units, and geographically. Job rotation is an uplifting process. We will be talking more about lateral movement in the future. In our recruiting at the MBA level, we are stressing more job rotation. That doesn't mean that you can't move up, but the process will be slower.

CHANGING MANAGERIAL ATTITUDES

> Success is a marathon, not a
> sprint.

Managers noted that companies will have to focus on employee and managerial performance and clearly define performance expectations. If something interferes with performance, is it the organization's job to solve the problem? Managers indicated that they can certainly make an array of tools available that will allow employees to solve problems on their own. They felt that employers must be ready to provide employees with the resources to overcome any barrier that is impairing the employee's ability to perform.

Mr. Spencer puts it this way:

> I want to provide the right counseling, the right backup support. If I have someone with a drug problem, I want to help. But if we can't, then that person ceases to be one of the right people for us. We are not in the rehabilitation business. We must deliver quality client services and make a profit.

The managers we interviewed recognized that even the best training and EAPs may have only a limited effect on employees. Senior managers, especially, noted that managers must understand the limitations of these programs and shouldn't feel disappointed either with themselves or with the employee if desired change is not always obtained. *Managers must recognize that change is not always going to come about even though there is a need for it.*

Management faces difficult challenges as we enter into a period of labor shortages and a likely reduction in the skill level of many new job entrants. The implementation of strong wellness/fitness programs can provide managers with powerful motivational tools—tools needed to keep their employees thinking positively and feeling well and fit. But the greatest challenge to managers, as individuals, will be to become truly concerned about their subordinates and fellow workers—to become truly caring people.

ENDNOTES

1. Cathy Trost, "Corporate Prenatal-Care Plans Multiply, Benefitting Both Mother and Employers," *The Wall Street Journal,* June 24, 1988, Sec. 2, p. 21.
2. Interview with Carl G. Sempier.
3. Interview with William P. Noyes.
4. Interview with William E. Spencer.
5. Interview with Raymond M. Fino.

SECTION 2

PROFILES OF AMERICA'S FITNESS/ WELLNESS PROGRAMS

Many companies, both large and small and in every sector of the business community, already have established fitness/wellness programs. The following descriptions of these programs provide excellent models for companies planning to start their own fitness/ wellness programs. The descriptions also provide an excellent opportunity for sharing ideas within the growing fitness/wellness movement.

AIR PRODUCTS AND CHEMICALS, INC.

Air Products and Chemicals, Inc. is engaged in the manufacture and marketing of industrial gases, chemicals, and cryogenic equipment and has major additional commitments in advanced materials and energy-related fields. The Company has 13,600 employees worldwide and has current annual sales revenues in excess of $2.5 billion.

Almost 4,000 employees are located at the Trexlertown (Allentown), Pennsylvania, headquarters. Management, research and administrative personnel comprise most of the population at this site. Major production facilities are located at Calvert City, KY; Pensacola, FL; Pasadena, TX; and Wilkes-Barre, PA. There are over 100 additional domestic production, distribution, and sales locations.

The Company has traditionally placed a very high value upon health, safety, and fitness and is active in all of these areas. Health promotion activities were initiated on a sustained basis in 1976 with programs in smoking cessation, nutrition and weight control, stress management, breast self-examination, and blood pressure screening.

The decision in 1985 to construct a Fitness Center in Allentown reflected the convergence of several influences. For years several hundred Company runners and joggers had used local roads and on-site trails that had been graded and surfaced. However, shower facilities were sharply limited. Similarly, various aerobic exercise classes had been offered for several years, but the continuous reassignment of available space for other purposes caused difficulties in offering a sustained program. Here, too, the lack of showers was a real problem.

In the early 1980s it had become a general feeling among most managers that fitness programs were becoming common among leading corporations whose judgments are carefully observed and considered by Air Products. A team of human resources, medical, and facilities services managers visited a number of existing corporate fitness facilities to assess programs,

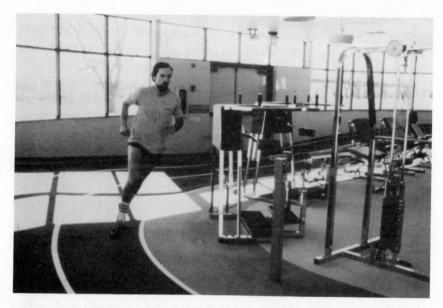

Fitness Center at Air Products and Chemicals, Allentown, Pennsylvania.

building design and construction, participant eligibility, staffing, and other operational issues. The decision to go forward with construction in 1985 reflected senior management's assessment of the worth of a fitness facility in promoting health, improving better integration of employees at all levels, providing a valid employee recruitment and retention tool, improving the quality of work life, and making a statement of Company values.

The 18,000-square-foot Fitness Center was completed in 1986. It features a 366 × 9-foot banked running track (14.4 laps/ mile) with a rubberized surface; men's and women's locker rooms, each with showers, dressing and grooming areas, whirlpool and sauna; and a group exercise room (2,300 sq. ft.). This multipurpose area is covered with resilient carpeting and is used for aerobics and other classes; the 28-foot ceiling height permits activities such as volleyball.

A full spectrum of exercise equipment is located within the running track perimeter. Included are Keiser muscular strength and endurance equipment, Biocycles, Air-Dyne and Bodyguard bicycle ergometers, Stairmasters, Concept II rowing machines, and Marquette treadmills. A wide range of group exercise classes are offered on a daily basis.

The Fitness Center staff includes four fitness professionals, a receptionist, and a maintenance-laundry worker. Additional part-time staff provide supplementary coverage. General custodial services are provided by the Company's site contractor.

The facility is open to Allentown employees from 6–9 A.M., 11 A.M.–1:30 P.M., and 4:30–8 P.M., with Saturday hours from 8 A.M.–12:30 P.M. Retirees may use the Center from 8:30–11:30 A.M.

Medical screening is required of all participants and consists of a health history questionnaire, a brief examination, determination of blood lipids and glucose, and an electrocardiogram. For persons age 40 or over or those with risk factors for coronary artery disease, a stress (treadmill) electrocardiogram is required and is conducted by the Company's medical staff.

Subsequent testing by the Center staff assesses the participant's current fitness level and leads to the development of personal fitness goals and exercise prescription. Testing includes measurements to determine body fat percentage (skinfold analysis), flexibility (sit and reach), and muscular strength and endurance (timed curl-ups, push-ups). All test information is entered into the Center's computer system, which allows the generation of a fitness profile, providing valuable feedback utilizing age and sex norms.

A $60 annual membership fee entitles participants to professional guidance, use of all facilities, towel service, and uniforms. Towels are laundered on-site as is exercise clothing contained for laundering in tagged nylon mesh bags.

Participants log in automatically using a bar-coded membership card. Mode, intensity, and duration of exercise are recorded by each participant at the end of the exercise period at one of several VDT keyboard stations. The system provides immediate feedback as to caloric equivalent of the exercise and integrates daily data into a monthly summary. A printout of the summary is mailed to each participant monthly. Participants can receive additional feedback through trending functions that plot calorie expenditure, body weight and participation over a specified period of time. The system allows various reports on program participation and facility utilization to be generated.

The Fitness Center is a focal point for various health promotion activities such as "Fats Off," a team weight loss competition; a prenatal health program; group walking competitions; and fun runs. A variety of other motivation and recognition programs, fitness challenges and special interest classes are also offered. A quarterly health promotion newsletter, group classes, and regular "lunch-n-learn" sessions are coordinated and implemented by a committee made up of members of the fitness, medical, and employee counseling staffs.

Air Products finds the Fitness Center to be an appropriate and valuable commitment to the enhancement of employee health and quality of work life. Whether or not similar but smaller scale programs can be implemented effectively at sites other than headquarters remains to be established, and several pilot efforts are now underway or proposed.

ARCO

ARCO, headquartered in Los Angeles, is one of the nation's leading oil companies. With a strong foundation in domestic crude oil and natural gas, ARCO is active in all phases of the petroleum industry: exploration, production, transportation and marketing. The company also mines and markets coal, manufactures and sells petrochemicals and has interests in solar energy. ARCO currently has more than 20,000 employees in various domestic and international locations.

Arco has always set its sights high, aiming to be a top performer in the industry. It is ARCO's employees who give the company its competitive edge. It is their imagination, risk-taking and creativity that help make ARCO a strong competitor. ARCO has a long-standing commitment to its employees' health and well-being, a commitment that has been demonstrated by its support of employee health programs.

ARCO's LIFELINE program provides an innovative approach that addresses personal welfare and longevity, as well as

Reprinted courtesy of ARCO.

human performance. This is accomplished through a personal Health Risk Assessment, which enables the employee to take direct responsibility for current health status. A monthly health newsletter complements the program. This voluntary program requires the employee to answer questions about personal habits and personal and family health background. In addition, serum cholesterol is obtained at the same time. The employee then receives a personalized report that compares him or her with norms established in a broad industrial population.

Future enhancement of this concept would include a cognitive profile that would also provide a personalized report to the employee about his or her verbal and spatial processing, logical thinking, frustration tolerance, dynamic memory and other measures relevant to cognitive (thinking) style.

The company pays the full cost of participation in LIFE-LINE. ARCO does not have access to the individual employee health status report. It is strictly confidential and sent directly by an independent contractor to the employee. However, the company does get an aggregate statistical report based on LIFELINE's findings, so that if there is a trend—for example, a high level of hypertension—ARCO can develop a program to alleviate the problem.

ARCO's Employee Assistance Program (EAP) has been a model for other companies aware of the need for professional intervention in the personal problems of employees. Company psychologists and a network of contract psychologists are available to provide prompt, professional counsel on a wide range of personal problems, with family and marital difficulties making up the largest share. The EAP Program has been available to ARCO employees since 1975 and has served more than 14,000 employees. Utilization of EAP has increased steadily over the years and the program now reaches over 6% of the employee population, a measure of the confidence employees have in the program.

A final link in ARCO's chain of employee health programs is the company's network of health care providers who favor prevention and an orientation to wellness. A significant effort to educate the employees is underway.

AT&T

AT&T's involvement in worksite disease prevention and health promotion dates back to the mid to late 70s when such activities were considered fads and perceived as add-ons to the traditional clinical services. Early activities included screenings, lunchtime health education series, health events and a few behavior-change interventions, such as smoking cessation, weight management and stress management. Interventions were offered as stand-alone programs, and there was little documentation of results, and follow-up was rare. However, these early efforts were successful to the extent that they set the stage for the future. Management was being educated about the benefits of health-promoting activities, employees were experiencing the personal merits of these preventive health services in the workplace and staff was building knowledge, skills, and expertise. It was because of this background that the Medical Department was prepared for the opportunity that was presented in the Spring of 1982.

TOTAL LIFE CONCEPT—THE EARLY STAGES OF DEVELOPMENT

Following the landmark Supreme Court decision announcing that AT&T would divest itself of its numerous operating companies, AT&T formed an inter-entity, interdepartmental Management of Change Committee. The charge to this committee was simple and complex at the same time. The challenge was to recommend strategies that would help the company and its then 1 million employees through a major reorganization not equal to anything that it had experienced in its 100 years of operation. The Medical Department recommended a Wellness Program. The original proposal was to conduct a pilot project and, based on the results of the

Reprinted courtesy of AT&T.

pilot, consider a companywide expansion. After several months of negotiation, a pilot was approved, and a pilot population of 2,000 AT&T employees, 1,000 each in Bedminster, N.J. and Kansas City, Mo. was selected. In addition, there were 1,250 employees selected as comparison subjects.

The study population received a Health Risk Appraisal and a follow-up panoply of programs to choose from while the comparison group received only the Health Risk Appraisal. At the end of one year the results demonstrated a positive impact and provided the impetus to the Medical Department to write another proposal, this one for nationwide expansion of the program.

TOTAL LIFE CONCEPT—EXPANSION

Throughout expansion, Total Life Concept adhered to the original model grounded in a mission statement that promised all employees an opportunity to pursue optimal well-being. Over the course of two and one half years, AT&T opened Fitness Centers and initiated individual health promotion programs in eight main regional locations from coast to coast. The original model was employee-focused, health/lifestyle module-oriented and completely staffed by full-time AT&T employees. It was a labor-intensive program, severely limited by the inability to reach all 300,000 employees located in some 1,600 locations. It was at the end of this initial expansion phase in mid-1987 that the delivery staffs became very aware of the gap between our mission and our capabilities under the existing client-centered, staff-intensive model.

TOTAL LIFE CONCEPT— A RECONCEPTUALIZATION

The mission and the focus of Total Life Concept (TLC) needed to change. If the program was to have a permanent place in the corporate structure, there needed to be a greater emphasis on organizational and environmental interventions; employees and managers needed a more prominent role and there needed to be greater emphasis placed on the use of vendors, community resources, and "suitcased" programs. A long redefinition process ensued during which the mission, goals, objectives, methods, and strategies were refined and organizational approval was obtained. Slowly, the Total Life Concept began to take on a new form as described in the following section.

TOTAL LIFE CONCEPT—A NEW BEGINNING

The newly defined TLC mission is to facilitate within AT&T a creative process for assessing, initiating and supporting positive health practices through organizational, individual, and environmental health promotion interventions. Three main program components exist, namely, Organizational, Individual and Environmental Health Promotion.

Organizational Health Promotion

The stated goal is to build a corporate culture that acknowledges the value of promoting optimal employee health as a primary business strategy. An assessment phase, the purpose of which is to gain insight into the organizational practices and norms which contribute to employee health and well-being, consists of management interviews, employee focus groups, an organizational survey and meetings with the union. Actual Organizational Health Promotion intervention begins when the commitment and interest of key managers has been established and the assessment phase is completed. A steering committee is then formed. This committee is responsible for making tactical decisions that will determine the scope and direction of the program.

The key component of Organizational Health Promotion is "Managing for Health." This seminar educates managers about the TLC process, increases their understanding of the health/productivity connection and guides them through a process of setting goals for personal and organizational health norm change. The theme throughout this seminar is to focus on the contributions that managers can make to self-esteem, well-being and performance capacity of work associates. Following "Managing for Health, " organizational representatives are selected to act as official health promotion liaisons. These representatives are specially trained by the TLC staff in order to prepare them for the duties and responsibilities connected with the implementation of TLC.

During the training, conceptual and theoretical information is presented as well as information about specific health risks. TLC activity and events are overviewed in detail. Without the ownership within the organization, promoting good health will never become an operational business strategy. It will merely be something that is talked about and not acted upon.

Individual Health Promotion (IHP)

Within the context of IHP, employees are provided with a wide range of opportunities to increase awareness of health risks and the health behaviors associated with these risks and are offered options for making health/lifestyle behavior change. Baseline assessment in the form of a health survey, a health risk appraisal and measurement of blood pressure, cholesterol, height and weight mark employees' entry into the process. A Wellness Planning Session is offered to provide a forum for individual health decision making where choices are made based on: (a) information from the Health Risk Appraisal Report, (b) motivation to change, (c) support for change, and (d) barriers to change. Following that session, employees are offered options for lifestyle improvement and health enhancement in the areas of:

Fitness	Back Care
Nutrition/Cholesterol	Blood Pressure Control
Weight Management	Smoking Cessation
Stress Management	Building Social Support

The behavior-change process is emphasized through classes, seminars, support groups and self-help.

Environmental Health Promotion (EHP)

EHP strives to establish a work environment that reflects AT&T's commitment to positive health. The objectives are: to make health fun, exciting and creative; promote events and activities that support good health practices; identify factors in the work environment that interfere with employees' ability to receive health-promoting messages, and provide an environment that complements the goals of individual lifestyle change efforts.

The major thrust of environmental support is to provide on-going program visibility that communicates healthy living at the worksite. The nature and extent of environmental health promotion is limited only by the creativity and energy of on-site staff and leaders.

A comprehensive overview of the program elements is provided in Tables 1, 2 and 3.

TABLE I
Total Life Concept (Organizational Health Promotion)

Assess	Initiate	Support
Management Interviews	Steering Committee—	Appraisal of Site
Focal Groups	strategic planning and	Coordinators and
Union Meeting	tactical decisions	Leadership Committee
Health Audit	Managing for Health I	Members based on
Disability Absence	Site Coordinator/	performance criteria
Incidental Absence	Leadership Committee	Follow-up Steering
Health Care Costs	Selection	Committee Meetings at
Medical Interviews	Site Coordinator/	12 month intervals
	Leadership Committee	Managing for Health II
	Training	Site Coordinator Trainings
		(as needed)

TABLE II
Total Life Concept (Individual Health Promotion)

Assess	Initiate	Support
Health Audit	Promotion Campaign	Support Groups
Health Risk Appraisal	"Life Choice" Process	Newsletter
(HRA)	Health Fair	Monthly Health
Serum Cholesterol	HRA	Campaigns
Blood Pressure	Wellness in Planning	Incentive Programs
Height	Session	Community Resources
Weight	Lifestyle Change	Medical/Clinical Support
Fitness Level	Categories	EAP Support
Weight Management	Fitness	
Nutrition	Nutrition	
Stress	Weight Management	
	Stress Management	
	Back Care	
	Blood Pressure Control	
	Smoking Cessation	
	Building Social Support	

TABLE III
Total Life Concept (Environmental Health Promotion)

Assess	Initiate	Support
Health Audit	Healthy Alternatives	Special Events
Safety Environment	Vending area	Contests
Toxic issues	Cafeteria	Promotional Activities
Ergonomic issues	Smoking Policy	
Cafeteria	Exercise Options	
Vending Areas	Changes in any	
Basic	environmental safety	
Light, heat, ventilation,	issues	
etc.		

CLOSING

While no longer a fad within AT&T or across business and industry, worksite health promotion is still growing rapidly and changing dramatically. National health concerns and, moreover, health care costs will continue to force an emphasis on health promotion and disease prevention. AT&T has come this far with a strong commitment to Total Life Concept and the current environment does not suggest that will change. The real challenge will be to continuously evolve as the nature of work, health and employment change.

BANK OF AMERICA

Bank of America is a financial services institution based in California, and with offices in several other major U.S. cities. It employs 55,000 employees who work in more than a thousand locales from branch offices to highrises.

Bank of America is committed to helping its employees live

healthy lifestyles. To assist in accomplishing this, a small unit was formed in 1983 called Corporate Health Programs, whose internal mission is to develop and implement employee health promotion programs. The objective is to enhance health and morale as well as, over time, limit medical plan and workers' compensation costs.

Corporate Health Programs staff consists of a manager and two health care professionals. Their expertise includes business/ marketing, public health, occupational health nursing and physical therapy.

Cost-effective programs have been developed that serve the diverse and widely scattered work settings of the bank's employees in an equitable way. The overall wellness program is called "Be Your Best." Under this banner are a series of programs that reach employees by newsletter, mail, video, and telephone.

ON YOUR BEHALF—PERSONNEL NEWS FOR BANK OF AMERICA EMPLOYEES

Corporate Health Programs has a section in this monthly publication. Starting in 1987 employees were introduced to a series of monthly challenges to improve their health in a simple, specific way. Challenges have included walking briskly at least four times a week for a minimum of 30 minutes each time, eating specific healthy foods daily, and completing a set of stretching exercises each day. Those employees completing the challenge and sending in a coupon from the newsletter were rewarded with one or more pamphlets that encourage good health practices. In addition, their coupon was put in a draw for 50 prizes each month which have included T-shirts, low-fat cookbooks, first aid kits and self-care books.

Along with the monthly challenge, there is a "By Request" section which offers specific materials at low or no cost on subjects such as smoking cessation, skin cancer, osteoporosis and AIDS. Both articles are very popular and employees frequently write in their appreciation for the support offered.

HYPERTENSION SELF-MANAGEMENT

This program is available on the request of a manager. The program comes in a kit, and includes information on the importance of the detection of hypertension, a digital blood pressure monitor, wall posters, a videocassette, and instructions on how to run the program. Employees who choose to participate send in their blood pressure readings to the registered nurse in Corporate Health Programs who screens each form and replies by letter to each one. Employees with elevated readings are contacted by phone and offered support in ways to lower their blood pressure. Everyone who participates receives a packet of helpful information on maintaining healthy lifestyles and is put on a mailing list to receive periodic mailings of supportive information.

AEROBICS

This program is available to managers whose employees express an interest in on-site aerobics exercise. It provides complete instruction for implementing a low-cost class including a survey of interest, room selection, criteria for selecting a qualified instructor, appropriate contract and release forms and information on the health benefits of aerobic exercise. To assist groups who may not have enough participants to sustain an instructor-led class, a videotape may be purchased at low cost from Corporate Health Programs, or they may use an audiotape or even be led by a qualified employee who volunteers to run a class.

HEALTH CLASSES

This program provides a framework for managers to access free health information classes from a variety of community resources. Brown bag lunches, or after-work sessions can be held on health subjects determined by a survey of employee interests. Health Maintenance Organizations, and agencies such as the American Cancer Society and the American Heart Association have speakers bureaus which will respond to requests.

HEALTH RESOURCES LIBRARY

A catalog of video and print materials on health and fitness is available to managers and employees. There are over thirty video titles, including several on self-help that may be borrowed for home watching. A deposit is requested for home videos which is returned to the borrower when the video is received by Corporate Health Programs. Some popular topics are back care, weight control, smoking cessation and stress management. There are over 100 titles in the print catalog which are free or low cost. Corporate Health Programs purchases carefully selected books in quantity at significant discounts and makes them available at low cost to the employees through the monthly newsletter. Books and materials are also available to our retirees.

STRESS MANAGEMENT

Corporate Health Programs conducts stress management classes at the request of managers. Also available to managers are a number of videos and booklets on managing stress that can be used individually or for a staff meeting discussion.

As time and money are a basic concern in any corporation, Corporate Health Programs constantly looks for high-impact, cost-effective and time-conserving programs that can bring the best health information to the employees of Bank of America.

BANK SOUTH CORPORATION

Bank South Corporation is a $4.1 billion-asset multibank holding company with headquarters in Atlanta. The bank opened in 1910 and has grown to become the third-largest Georgia-based financial institution.

Bank South is a statewide organization with over 120 offices

Reprinted courtesy of Bank South Corporation.

Bank South Corporate Philosophy

	We at Bank South share this philosophy expressing our values, beliefs, expectations and guiding principles. The philosophy sets high standards of excellence for ourselves as a company, as bankers, and as individuals.
Customer Orientation	We will be sensitive to the needs and expectations of our customers, recognizing that we exist and prosper because of them.
Quality	We will measure everything that represents us—people, services, facilities, systems, training—by the highest standards of quality.
Professionalism	We will be thoroughly trained in technical and specialized areas of banking and finance as well as in human relations. Our managers will be people-oriented and visible and accessible to all our people at all levels of the company.
Fiscal Health	We will manage for the long term, always keeping in mind the importance of economic growth, financial soundness, and profitability.
Planning	We will have a clearly defined plan against which opportunities and issues may be evaluated, decisions made, and responsibilities understood and communicated throughout the company.
Open Communications	We will share information broadly in an attempt to keep our people as informed as possible on our plans, opportunities, problems and progress.
Team Approach	We will accomplish our corporate goals by working together and by practicing participative management. We will work to promote the company as a whole and not groups or individuals.
Career Development	We will attract, train, motivate and retain quality people, and our compensation programs will reflect high expectations for superior performance. We will provide equal employment opportunities for all our people to build careers rather than just jobs. We recognize our people as our most important asset.
Risk Management not Risk Avoidance	We will encourage innovation and action-oriented decision-making, as our mission is to succeed, rather than to try not to fail.
Ethical and Moral Values	We will set and follow the highest ethical and moral standards as a company and as individuals.
Civic Involvement	The communities we serve are our livelihood and we have a responsibility as a company and as individuals to be good, solid, active citizens.
Fun and Excitement	Our careers at Bank South should be enjoyable and exciting, and they will be as we practice this philosophy.

in 23 counties and 43 municipalities throughout Georgia. This compares to 42 offices in four counties and 13 municipalities in 1980. Bank South added 42 offices during 1987, primarily in metropolitan Atlanta, where the bank now has 86 offices and over 2,500 employees. Many of these are open until 8:00 P.M., six days a week, conveniently located inside Kroger and Ingles supermarkets.

Prosperity has accompanied this rapid growth. Earnings have increased from $10 million in 1980 to $27 million in 1987. *Forbes* magazine has listed Bank South as one of 300 "Up and Coming" companies in the country and also as one of the nation's top 400 companies in assets. *Business Week* magazine includes Bank South among the 1,000 most valuable companies in America.

Programs currently offered at Bank South include a Fitness Seminar which consists of blood lipid profiles, a fitness test, resting EKG, individual exercise prescriptions and weekly lectures on various health and fitness topics. The Nutrition Seminar consists of blood lipid profiles, body fat measurements, and individual dietary analysis and prescriptions in addition to weekly lectures on nutrition. All tests are re-done at the end of the seminar. Additionally, we offer Smoking Cessation on a regular basis and aerobics four nights a week at the four location in the Metro Atlanta area, as well as at three community banks. Health Screens such as Diabetes, Blood Pressure and Glaucoma are also held every other month as well as "Lunchbox Lectures," which are free of charge and available to all employees.

Branch and community wellness programs are scheduled on a monthly basis. Other plans include the implementation of a smoke-free environment by November 16, 1989, concurrent with the "Great American Smokeout."

Outside specialists such as exercise physiologists and dietitians are contracted to do most of the programs. United Way at Work is also used extensively.

New employees are made aware of the "Fulltime Good Health" schedule and philosophy in the orientation meeting, which is held on a weekly basis.

The Incentive Program at Bank South helps keep employees motivated. "Fulltime Good Health" bucks are earned for participating in the various wellness programs as well as for verifiable outside aerobic activities. The points are redeemed for prizes such as shirts, shorts, athletic bags, lunch cooler bags and t-shirts with the "Fulltime Fitness" Logo on them. In addition, gift certificates from Champ's Sporting Goods which can be redeemed for $25 of miscellaneous goods or $55-$65 coupons for walking shoes, running shoes, and aerobic shoes are currently available.

BP AMERICA, INC.

Less than two years ago, the Standard Oil Company, the original Rockefeller Standard, merged with the U.S. operations of the British Petroleum Company, p.l.c. (BP). Now BP America (BPA), we are the 12th largest industrial company in the U.S. and the world's third largest oil company.

BP America is comprised of companies under the following businesses: oil and gas exploration and production; crude oil and petroleum products; transportation; refining and marketing; minerals and precious metals; chemicals; coal; nutrition; computer software; and industrial products. BP America has locations across the United States and Canada. BPA presently employs approximately 40,000 employees.

Currently BPA operates its own fitness centers in Cleveland, Ohio; Lima, Ohio; Houston, Texas; and Anchorage, Alaska. Our businesses also subsidize the cost of local exercise facilities for employees in Dayton and Toledo, Ohio; Niagara Falls, New York; and New Carlisle, Indiana where there are no on-site facilities.

The largest fitness center is located in the BPA Headquarters building in Cleveland, Ohio. The facility covers 15,000 square feet and consists of a reception area, staff offices, exercise equipment room, aerobics room, lockers and shower facilities. A professional exercise physiology staff consisting of a Ph.D., M.Ed., and M.A. oversee the facility and related activities.

Reprinted courtesy of BP America, Inc.

The fitness center is open from 6:15 A.M. until 7:00 P.M. Monday through Friday, making it convenient for all levels of employees to use the center. All full-time BPA employees who have had a fitness evaluation are eligible to use the fitness center free of charge. In the exercise equipment room, employees can pedal stationary bicycles including the popular Lifecycles, run or walk on motorized and manual treadmills, row on two different kinds of stationary rowing machines, "ski cross-country" on Nordic ski machines or climb stairs on our newest addition to the fitness center, the Stairmaster 4000. Employees also have the option to build strength on Kaiser Cam II weight training machines, which operate on pneumatic resistance, or use the free weights. In total, there are over 40 pieces of equipment available.

In the aerobics room, employees can participate in a number of scheduled group activities, such as aerobic dance or calisthenics. Presently, there are 11 different types of aerobic programs offered which vary in intensity and activity. Along with the traditional aerobic dance classes, we also offer a pregnancy class and a sports conditioning class. Classes are conducted Monday through Friday mornings, lunch hours and evenings. One wall of the aerobics room is covered with mirrors so that participants can check their body alignment while exercising. The floor provides a flexible surface for injury prevention. All instructors are aerobic-certified as well as CPR-certified.

Employees have the ability to log their activities and exercise level through the Fitness Center computer system using HMC software. By completing this process, employees receive a written summary of their monthly accomplishments, including calories burned and aerobic points earned. Currently, we have two programs which award employees for their efforts. At the end of each month we compile the exercise data and award "sport-leader" t-shirts to the top three males and females in each of many categories including calories burned, aerobic points, treadmill time, walk/jog time, aerobic class time, and so on. Also, this year beginning in January, we initiated our "Consistency Recognition Program" (CRP). CRP is a program in which employees are recognized for their consistency in achieving 12 visits a month to the fitness center. Employees can earn four different gift items, in succession, based on computerized logging of their activities and achieving 12 visits a month. To earn all four gift items, the employee must consistently exercise 12 times a month for a period of 10 months (the 10 months do not have to be consecutive). These two programs have been very successful in increasing fitness center use and use of the computer for logging in fitness activities. Feedback from employees regarding the CRP has been extremely positive and for those once-inconsistent exercisers, the programs offer a positive and worthwhile challenge to become consistent.

Approximately 30 percent of BPA's 2,500 Headquarters employees use the center regularly, and nearly all Headquarters employees have completed the comprehensive fitness evaluation required prior to using the facility. This evaluation includes health background and dietary information as well as a battery of other tests including body composition measures, heart rate, blood pressure, cardiovascular fitness (determined through a submaximal bicycle test while connected to an electrocardiogram machine), flexibility, and muscular strength and endurance. All results are discussed with the employee during a consultation which is scheduled at the time of the evaluation. An exercise prescription is then designed by the exercise specialists tailored for the employee's individual needs. The modern equipment, professional staff, convenient hours, attractive surroundings, lockers and shower facilities make the fitness center easy to use.

HELP YOURSELF TO HEALTH PROGRAM

BPA's National Health and Fitness Program's philosophy is to assist employees in obtaining optimal health through health awareness, health education, health risk reduction, behavior modification and physical activity.

Health awareness attempts to increase employee awareness of the importance of maintaining a healthy lifestyle and to motivate them to take steps to improve their health. This is achieved through our strong support for community events such as the Great American Smokeout, Heart Disease and Cancer Awareness Months, the March of Dimes WalkAmerica, Cystic Fibrosis Sports Challenge, Revco Cleveland Marathon and many more. BPA's

Health and Fitness staff also monitor health topics and issues in the media and transfer these into corporate acceptance.

Health education provides the employees with information regarding which lifestyle changes should and could be made, and how to achieve these changes. Employees are provided with current information on major topics such as nutrition, exercise, AIDS, cancer, medical self-exams, mental health and more. We have an ongoing program entitled "Help Yourself to Health." This program helps educate our employees and their families through BPA's Corporate Health Newsletter—a monthly publication reaching the homes of 22,000 employees; lunchtime health education seminars; a Health and Fitness Center newsletter, distributed in-house; ongoing health speakers bureaus; "Ask the Expert," which is a question and answer session; Women's Health Series, a videotape library available to all employees to check out videotapes on health and related issues; and brochures on nearly all health concerns.

Behavior modification involves programs aimed at modifying unhealthy behavior. On-site behavioral modification programs include smoking cessation, weight reduction, stress management, nutritional analysis and counseling, and participation in our athletic clubs (i.e. runners' club, walkers' club and cyclists' club). The programs are operated by our own staff and facilitate lifestyle changes through convenience, consistency and follow-up. The convenience of our quality exercise and aerobics facility has helped many employees to begin a regular exercise schedule to improve their cardiovascular fitness.

Most health risks are identified by the medical and nursing staff of the Company's Occupational Health Clinic allowing the Health and Fitness staff to cooperatively assist the medical professionals in counseling employees through on-site health risk reduction programs. Health risk reduction programs are formal health screening programs used to help employees voluntarily identify if they are at risk for medical illness and disease. We can then either provide treatment through a health program, or direct the employee to proper community medical resources. These screenings include blood pressure, elevated cholesterol, and glaucoma, to name a few. BPA's health risk reduction programs also include after-hours, on-premises support groups. These were formed for employees coping with stressful situations who might benefit by support from others with like illnesses or problems. This past year, an Alzheimer's Disease Support Group was established for employees, spouses, parents or relatives with Alzheimer's Disease or related disorders. Future plans include support groups for adult children of alcoholics, post-heart attack patients, cancer patients and asthmatics.

BPA has established expertise in health education and fitness and is now recognized as an industry leader in this area. BPA's Corporate Health, Safety and Environmental Quality Department continues its efforts to establish these programs in all major BPA locations around the country, through on-site consultation and training programs. Finally, we would like to expand these programs to other companies within the BP international group.

CENTRAL STATES HEALTH & LIFE CO. OF OMAHA

For Central States Health & Life Co. of Omaha (CSO), the momentum just keeps building as an already progressive health promotion program becomes even stronger. Management's attitude toward worksite wellness is reflected in its continuing commitment to creating a healthy workplace.

Over the years, Central States has been known in the insurance industry, in the community, and across the country as a leader in wellness. Due in large part to the passionate commitment of its progressive chairman, the company has become a "well new workplace" and model for companies everywhere.

With the guidance of an all-employee advisory committee, CSO's chairman has put into practice company policies that reflect corporate concern for health, wellness, and the family.

Reprinted courtesy of Central States Health & Life Co. of Omaha.

ORGANIZATIONAL SETTING

Central States Health & Life Co. is an insurance company specializing in individual health and life, credit, and credit-card life, disability, and unemployment plans. The Home Office is located on an expansive suburban tract in Omaha, Neb., on which the company has built an outdoor running track and exercise course.

Of the nearly 500 employees, 72 percent are women and 28 percent men, with an average age of 32. The company is largely clerical and professional. As is common in the insurance industry nationwide, the typical employee is a working woman with pre-school-age children. She holds a clerical position with an average salary of $791 per month. Because women are disproportionately represented among employee ranks, the wellness programming focuses on many issues of particular interest to women such as women's health, prenatal care, osteoporosis, and child care.

As an insurance company, CSO exists to help people minimize financial risk by offering quality insurance products. At the same time, the company perceives its mission to "encourage people to take responsibility for their own health and to make wellness a way of living a longer, healthier life."

CSO's involvement in wellness began with its current chairman and CEO, William McBain Kizer. Over 20 years ago, Mr. Kizer sat down with auditors in the claims department and asked why so many people were in the hospital or had died. To him, it seemed as if their illnesses had been caused by their own lifestyles. Many of them smoked, ate and drank too much, and didn't pay attention to their health. Research has since proven that Mr. Kizer's assumptions years ago are indeed true: Half the people in the hospital are there because of their own lifestyle-induced habits.

Mr. Kizer knew he couldn't do anything about the health of his company's policyholders, but he knew he could do something about his own health and the health of his employees.

In 1976 when the new Home Office was constructed, wellness in the form of exercise equipment and a locker room was offered as an executive park at CSO for men only. Locker rooms and exercise equipment for women were added a few years later, and both facilities were open to all employees.

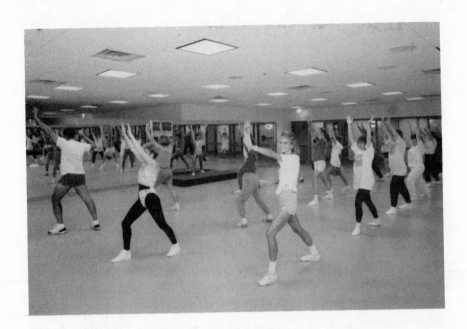

CONTINUING COMMITMENT TO WELLNESS

Completed in 1988, a five-story addition to the Home Office contains an expansive aerobic room and two equipment rooms alongside larger men's and women's locker and shower facilities.

Staffing for CSO's wellness program includes a full-time and a part-time wellness director. Today they oversee a wellness program that would be considered ambitious in any size company.

Briefly, CSO's approach to wellness concentrates on smoking, alcohol use, nutrition, exercise, and health education. These components are part of Mr. Kizer's SANE approach to creating a healthy workplace (S for smoking, A for alcohol, N for nutrition, and E for exercise) introduced in his book *The Healthy Workplace: A Blueprint for Corporate Action* (published by John Wiley & Sons, 1987).

Smoking: As an extension of the company's long-term commitment to creating a healthy workplace, CSO entered 1988 with a smoke-free environment. Employees are periodically offered subsidized stop-smoking classes.

Alcohol: The company has a written policy on alcohol use at company-sponsored events. In short, the policy states that nonalcoholic beverages are to be prominently displayed along with their alcoholic counterparts. In conjunction with the alcohol policy, the company urges, through a written policy, that employees wear seat belts at all times (seat belt use is required in all company-owned cars).

Nutrition: CSO's cafeteria offers healthful choices in the company cafeteria. An outside food service is required to post calories and maintain an attractive and inexpensive salad bar. Subsidized weight management classes are offered, as are periodic cholesterol and blood sugar screenings. Blood pressure testing is available at any time during the workday.

Exercise: In addition to individual workout equipment, aerobics are conducted during the lunch hour and after work. And classes in stress reduction are offered regularly by the company's training department. Monthly brown-bag lunch sessions are held, and guest speakers present informative talks on health issues.

One particular health issue at Central States involves maternal and infant health. Because so many staff members are young women of child-bearing age, the wellness staff regularly conducts an educational series about pregnancy, childbirth, and newborn care, with help from the March of Dimes. Pregnant employees receive a packet of brochures and discounts on "baby items." And mothers-to-be who refrain from smoking and drinking during their pregnancy receive a $50 savings bond for the newborn infant.

Employees are allowed work time off and are encouraged to attend annual health fairs conducted in the company's offices. The health fair offers several health screenings, and the company subsidizes the cost for employees and their family members who wish to have blood drawn at the health fair for full laboratory testing. Confidential results are sent directly to employees at their homes.

All the components of a strong health promotion program set the stage for the development of innovative incentive programs at CSO. Cash and prizes are awarded for participants in "Go for the Gold," "Holiday Health," "Wheel of Wellness," and "Ticket to Wellness."

Because years ago Mr. Kizer recognized the importance of human capital, he actively initiated wellness within his company and encouraged private sector initiatives to promote worksite wellness throughout the United States. These efforts have helped to establish the Wellness Council of the Midlands (WELCOM) in Omaha, of which Mr. Kizer is a founder. Cities across the country adopted the WELCOM model in forming their own Wellness Councils, with help from the Health Insurance Association of America.

In 1987, Mr. Kizer led the formation of a national nonprofit umbrella organization known as the Wellness Councils of America (WELCOA) to further help establish Wellness Councils in cities everywhere.

PROGRAM RATIONALE

Participation in CSO's wellness programs is voluntary. Management support is in place, as is the company's flex-time policy. Generally, employees find it easy to rearrange their workday to accommodate a lunchtime speaker or to fit in an aerobic workout. Most activities are free to the employees.

RESULTS

CSO's turnover rate is significantly below average for the insurance industry. The vice-president of personnel attributes lower staff turnover to increased employee morale as a result of the emphasis on employee welfare and wellness. Through this emphasis,

CSO is serving as a model and setting an example for other insurance companies. Informal studies reveal lower health insurance claims and fewer sick days used by active participants in wellness programs when compared with a group of employees who never take part.

A comment on the nonparticipants in any wellness activities: Even though the company offers flex hours, many of the young working mothers feel particularly time pressured during their workday—and may not participate as actively as they would like. But when a company like CSO creates a healthy workplace, these employees too are part of the larger healthy picture. They eat lunch in a cafeteria where they can make nutritious choices; they work in a smoke-free environment; and they work with other well people. Certainly that corporate culture claims a 100 percent participation rate.

CHAMPION INTERNATIONAL CORPORATION

Champion International Corporation, a paper and forest products company with 23,000 domestic employees, has a company-wide wellness initiative called the Champions for Life Health and Fitness Program. The program is an integral part of the Champion culture and is continuing to prosper as it expands to more locations. A review of how the program got started and evolved into a part of the corporate business strategy tells a lot about the program, and the company.

Beginning as an exercise program for corporate headquarters employees in 1981, the program quickly made the transition to a comprehensive wellness program. In 1983, the enlightened C.E.O. understood the impact a healthier, more productive workforce would have on the company's bottom line. Senior management saw the potential of bringing the program to all of its locations, but did not know how to engineer it. This created a window of opportunity for the health and fitness department's professionals.

Their objective was clear. They needed to create a health and fitness system which would attract participation while promoting interest and support. The program was designed to meet and exceed professional standards for such programs. Another objective was to be able to show senior management and the rest of the company a significant return on their investment. The staff needed to establish a credible program that worked.

Champion's health and fitness program is an integral part of the company's overall business strategy. The company's goal is to be in the top quartile of American industry and attain a 15–16% return on equity (R.O.E.). The health and fitness program's role, as part of this informal cost control team, is to have a positive impact on productivity and absenteeism. At the same time, it is hoped that medical claims and workers' compensation costs will be reduced. In addition, the program enhances employee retention and recruitment. Lastly, the program works to improve and complement the work environment at Champion.

Champion is currently about one-third of the way into the ever-evolving participative management culture. In this environment, decision making is pushed down to the lowest level possible. Employees have a much greater say in how they are doing their jobs. The health and fitness program serves as a tangible example of participative management.

First, individuals have the opportunity to take more control of their lifestyles because they now have the health information to make wise choices for themselves. In addition, employees assist in program development by providing input through health and fitness advisory committees.

The health and fitness staffs at various locations work with other departments to provide a healthy work environment. The development of a corporate-wide smoking policy and smoking cessation health education material is producing a very positive impact. Healthy nutritional choices are offered in both the cafeteria and vending areas. Safety issues such as work shoe/foot care and back problems are addressed also. Lastly, a major emphasis of programming includes family involvement. Through the collective efforts of many employees at the various locations, the work environment is becoming healthier and more efficient.

In order to display its role in Champion's business strategy, evaluation systems are in place to determine program efficacy. The program is viewed as being on a continuum. Evaluation is on-going in different ways at appropriate stages along the continuum. Laurels are not thought about; they simply do not exist.

Ongoing evaluation allows the department to keep tabs on the progress being made. Participation and physiological data are tracked, compared and contrasted among the locations. For example, the exercise facilities use a software package, Champion Health Assessment Program (CHAP) to monitor physiological profiles, health risks and exercise workouts of the participants. Health education participation and health screening results are evaluated and communicated to employees and management.

Formalized studies assist the staff in stepping back from their efforts to take a look at hard data such as medical claims, absenteeism and employees' attitudes and perceptions of the program. The studies enable the staff to support its role in the business strategy. They also allow the staff to re-evaluate its philosophy and systems, be responsive to changes within Champion and, ultimately, insure continued growth.

The Champion health and fitness department provides programming to its employees, retirees, and spouses. The wide range of voluntary health enhancement efforts are comprised of four components: health assessment, health education, medical self-care, and exercise programs.

The health assessment component is designed to help individuals discover where they stand in various health areas. Examples include blood pressure and cholesterol screenings, health risk appraisals and physiological profiles. They help individuals to tailor the health program to their needs.

Health education involves providing the information employees need to assume personal responsibility for their health and well-being. Examples of the topics are: nutrition, smoking cessation, weight management, cancer prevention, stress management, back care, and CPR. These topics are communicated using different mediums and incorporating innovative means in order to educate.

The third component is medical self-care. The emphasis here is to help individuals become wise consumers of medical services. Asking intelligent questions of doctors, knowing where to go for particular medical care, the use of generic drugs and the benefits of same day surgery are some of the topics addressed.

Exercise programs, both individualized and group, promote regular exercise among employees, retirees and spouses. Combined with other positive health behaviors, exercise serves to reduce the risk of heart disease and improve cardiovascular health. Larger company locations have on-site exercise facilities, while others may provide partially subsidized memberships at selected community fitness centers. In addition, company-wide exercise promotions such as the Turkey Trot Marathon and Heart Throb foster camaraderie, involve the family, and are just good fun.

The combined effects of the four program components assist individuals in leading healthier, more productive lives. The guiding philosophy is that people want to stay well and will do so if they have the information and the means to carry out a successful wellness program.

Champion International Corporation is strongly committed to the ideal that the employee is its most valuable resource. In a competitive global economy, the human resources of a company will be the deciding factor in determining who is most profitable. The Champions for Life Health and Fitness Program will continue to evolve and grow. In this way, it will play a significant role in Champion reaching its business goals.

CHRYSLER CORPORATION

Chrysler Corporation is a diversified multi-billion dollar company involved in automotive and aircraft manufacturing, electronics and financial services. The company, which is headquartered in Highland Park, Michigan and has 150,000 employees worldwide, consists of three separate operating groups: Chrysler Motors, Chrysler Financial and Chrysler Technologies.

Keeping pace with a rapidly changing world and economic climate requires that Chrysler meet new demands squarely.

Reprinted courtesy of Chrysler Motors Corporation and Valerie A. Brannas, M.S.W.

Thus, the corporate credo of "Teaming Up To Be The Best" has meant reaching out to the collective intelligence and spirit of our employees to be able to produce affordable, high quality and on-target products and services. Our internal climate clearly is changing to better accommodate and utilize our vast human resources.

Employee health and wellness is one extension of that phenomena. Other features are increased cooperation and joint activities shared by the corporation and the primary union, the International Union, United Automobile, Aerospace and Agricultural Implement Workers of America, UAW. Revolutionary "Modern Operating Agreements" promise to create participatory employee atmospheres unsurpassed in any Big Three auto plant with decision-making shared in many new areas. The UAW-Chrysler National Training Center administers major employee programs and provides worksite training and employee development courses across the corporation. Also, a primary focus on quality improvement is helping to propel changes internally, as well as in our most visible products—our cars and trucks.

A new and expanded Employee Assistance Program (EAP) was launched in 1988, providing for the first time full-time EAP representatives in 46 of our plants and facilities. With the professional back-up of a national network, EAP reps touch the lives of thousands of Chrysler employees, with information and direct support, contributing to a well workforce.

Health promotion is just a part of a bigger picture. In 1984, Chrysler began it's pilot health program at one of it's machining plants by contracting with Control Data Corporation for the StayWell program. Since that time, programs have begun at several additional plant sites and the corporate headquarters. Through these programs, Chrysler and the UAW are working to help employees and their families reduce lifestyle health risks through health screenings, education and support. Control Data, by contracting with local hospitals to provide on-site program management, ensures that these educational and assessment features are conducted by highly qualified nurses and health education professionals.

Although health screenings are paid for entirely by the corporation, course fees are split by the employee and company with an additional incentive rebate going to employees who complete a course. Other StayWell activities have been offered at minimal or no cost. These activities have included special events such as exercise equipment demonstrations, low calorie snack samples and health cooking tips. Action teams, groups of employees who share a common health-related interest, are formed to encourage and support members. The main risk areas addressed by StayWell are smoking, exercise, weight, nutrition and stress. The corporation committed to institute a restrictive smoking policy in 1988–1989 with smoking cessation courses to be offered corporate-wide to employees who opt to quit.

The wellness program features have been evolving too, making changes as we better learn how to provide attractive, enjoyable and effective programming. At one site, employees who voluntarily sign a release form at the time of screening and who are found to be "at risk" for one of several cardiovascular-related health risks are contacted by the hospital and invited to participate in a mini-course on that risk area. In addition, a variety of new materials and formats are being tested at several sites with the objective of providing bite-sized activities and better ways to fit wellness activities into already busy schedules. Examples are the introduction of mini-courses along with the regular length courses, and an eight-week, incentive-based home exercise program involving the awarding of prizes to employees who meet a given level of exercise, as well as the normal aerobics classes. At our sprawling world headquarters in Highland Park, communication and participation are enhanced by a growing network of "delegates" from each department, providing fresh apples to employees to encourage them to sign up for the free Health Risk Appraisal and Screening. Several hundred such delegates are helping to spread the word.

The new Chrysler Technology Center, now under construction in Auburn Hills, Michigan, will feature a fully equipped and professionally staffed fitness center when it opens in the early 1990s. High participation and overall fitness, aimed at cardiovascular risk reduction, are important objectives. The center will be carefully evaluated to determine whether fitness centers are to be installed at other sites.

Experience has taught us that it is not a simple thing to effectively promote wellness. It takes money, creativity and lots of hard work. We find ourselves in a unique place in history where companies are rapidly becoming a major source of health education for their employees, and ultimately, within their communities. Chrysler is proud to be making its contribution.

THE CIGNA COMPANIES

The CIGNA companies are leading providers of insurance, health care, employee benefits and related financial services to businesses and individuals worldwide. With headquarters in Philadelphia, the companies had assets of more than $55 billion at year-end 1988 and employed more than 48,000 people.

The Corporate Medical Department started the Preventive Medical Program at the Philadelphia headquarters in 1979 to help prevent employee heart disease and sedentary lifestyle disorders. Its main objectives are to (1) identify risk factors through preventive medical screening and (2) facilitate healthy lifestyle changes by educating and motivating employees to reduce risk behaviors and optimize their health and fitness.

To identify risk factors, all employees are offered periodic health examinations based on their age. The exam routinely includes a thorough physician's examination, a review of the medical history, an appraisal of health risks, and the following tests: body composition analysis, muscle strength, lower back flexibility, exercise tolerance, pulmonary function, resting ECG, blood lipid profile, blood count, urinalysis, hemoccult, visual acuity and tonometry. If medically indicated, the exam may also include proctosigmoidoscopy, gynecological examination, chest x-ray and a maximal ECG stress test.

A staff physician and an exercise physiologist/health educator then provide a follow-up consultation to clarify existing risk factors, jointly establish health goals with the employee and implement appropriate intervention strategies.

Employees are encouraged to participate in appropriate ongoing wellness programs such as stress management, smoking

---

cessation, cholesterol screening, mammography, low back school, aerobic exercise classes, blood pressure screening, weight-loss programs, corporate running programs, CPR training and others.

In most cases, the intervention strategies also will include physical activities to develop cardiovascular fitness and improve muscle tone and flexibility. The exercise physiologist develops an individualized exercise program based on the employee's exercise preferences, history and current fitness level.

Employees have access to the 7,000 square-foot Corporate Fitness Center to pursue their exercise programs. The facility is professionally staffed with exercise physiologists and specialists, who closely monitor all programs and provide participants with regular feedback and personalized information.

The Fitness Center equipment includes nine motorized treadmills for running and walking, 15 stationary bicycle ergometers, three rowing machines, two stair-climbing machines, a cross-country skier, an upper body ergometer, nine Nautilus weight machines and assorted dumbbells.

The staff operates the center 12 hours daily and provides exercise clothing and towels to make its facilities as accessible as possible. A quarterly "Fit to Print" newsletter, monthly phone calls, memo reminders and frequent motivational incentive programs encourage the well-intentioned employee to exercise regularly.

Employees share the costs of the Fitness Center by contributing $208 annually for membership privileges. In its 10 years of operation, the number of employees using the center has increased every year.

The effectiveness of the Preventive Medical Program has been demonstrated by comprehensive individual and group statistical reports, prepared with computer analysis of medical, exercise and attendance data. These evaluations have helped document the medical benefits of regular participation at the Fitness Center, substantiating the strong correlation between the frequency of exercise and the health of the employee. Personal case histories and testimonials add qualitative proof of the program's success.

In the future, the Preventive Medical Program will expand the spectrum of health and wellness programs to meet the needs of all CIGNA company employees worldwide. Plans are underway for a comprehensive 15,000-square-foot Wellness Center in the new offices to open in 1991 in Philadelphia.

COLONIAL LIFE & ACCIDENT INSURANCE COMPANY

Colonial Life & Accident Insurance Company specializes in supplemental and basic insurance products sold on an individual basis through payroll deduction to employees and managers at their place of employment. Nearly 1,000 employees work at the company's home office in Columbia, South Carolina.

Colonial is a high-volume, high-performance company, and management believes that corporate success depends on employees who enjoy their work and make positive contributions to the overall productivity of the company. Colonial expects a great deal from employees, most of whom work at video display terminals. Many interact with clients over the telephone, and they must be able to respond to customer requests courteously, quickly and accurately. For several years, management has recognized the need for systematic ways to help relieve employees' stress and increase their levels of concentration and productivity.

One method of addressing this issue is the corporate wellness program, "Time Out For Life," which was introduced in 1983 and has evolved into a model for employer-sponsored health promotion programs. In 1985 it received the Governor's Worksite Health Promotion Award for the best program in the State of South Carolina.

Colonial's on-site fitness center offers a complete set of Eagle weight-training equipment, stationary bicycles, treadmills, slantboards, an exercise area with a Spring-Aire aerobics floor where classes are conducted, men's and women's locker and shower rooms complete with hair dryers, and laundry facilities. The center is open from 7 A.M. to 7 P.M. every workday, and employees are encouraged to exercise before and after work and dur-

---

Reprinted courtesy of Colonial Life & Accident Insurance Co.

ing their lunch breaks. Colonial's flex-time system makes it easy for employees to fit exercising into their daily schedules.

Fifteen exercise classes, led by a staff of part-time certified instructors, are conducted each week in the fitness center. Classes are offered at 7:15 A.M., 12:10 P.M., 4:15 P.M. and 5:15 P.M., and include low-impact, regular and "challenger" aerobics and conditioning classes. Other classes conducted on-site have included yoga, ballet and modern dance.

Some classes are conducted off-site at local parks and recreation centers. In 1988 these included beginning and intermediate racquetball, beginner and intermediate tennis, and water aerobics.

As of January 1987, new employees are required to have a health consultation, and all employees are encouraged to participate in an annual consultation on a voluntary basis. The health consultation includes a lifestyle analysis, bloodwork, fitness assessment (which includes a stress test, percentage of body fat, blood pressure, vision check and flexibility test) and physician screening. The objectives of the health consultation are to assess the employee's current health status, identify possible risk factors, and suggest an intervention program. The health consultation is a condition of employment, but it is conducted after an employee is hired and has no impact on an individual's employment status.

To participate in any Time Out For Life exercise program employees must be approved through the health consultation or have the written consent of a doctor. Spouses may also join. Membership fees are nominal and payable by payroll deduction, and new members are asked to attend a brief orientation.

Other components of Time Out For Life are free lunchtime and after-work programs on health education topics, including an ongoing self-hypnosis clinic, first aid and CPR training, stress management, smoking cessation, weight control, and lectures on subjects such as diabetes, back pain, mammography, working at the VDT, parenting, cholesterol, sports injuries and household safety. The company cafeteria and breakrooms provide a selection of low-calorie foods prepared in accordance with American Heart Association dietary guidelines. A program director and two full-time exercise physiologists assist employees with their personal wellness programs.

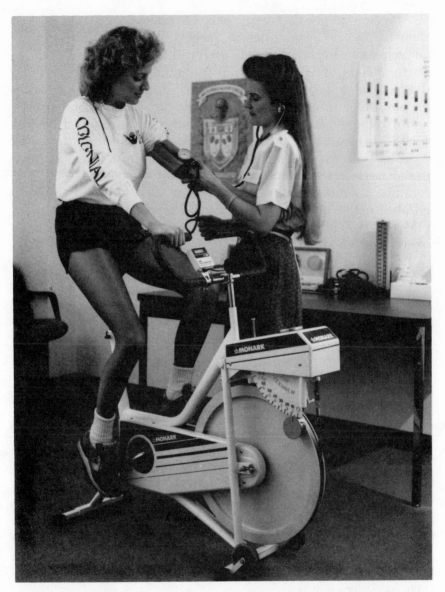

Checking blood pressure after workout at Colonial Life Insurance Company. (*Michael Moore*)

Since employees are being asked to make positive changes in their lifestyles, Colonial has an incentive program to encourage participation. Each activity is assigned a specific number of incentive points, and employees can accumulate points by exercising (both at the wellness center and on their own), by participating in classes, and by practicing healthy behaviors, such as not drinking and driving. These incentive points are then exchanged for gift certificates from a local sporting goods store.

Wellness has become part of the corporate culture at Colonial. There is a no-smoking policy in all work areas, and it is common to see employees putting on their athletic shoes to climb stairs or walk during their breaks, selecting the "wellness plate" in the cafeteria, and heading toward the fitness center to exercise after work.

Employees have responded enthusiastically to Time Out For Life, and management is pleased with the participation rate. The first year of the program, when health consultations were voluntary, 89.9 percent of the employees had a health consultation, and in 1987 nearly half of the population participated in a voluntary re-screening. In 1987, 556 employees—well over half of the total population—completed enough wellness activities to earn incentive gifts.

Management believes that the program has been a sound investment, although there has been no attempt to collect any data to substantiate this belief. The Chairman of the Board, Gayle O. Averyt, is so committed to the concept of worksite health promotion that he recently spearheaded a movement to form a wellness council in Columbia. WELCOM SC, the Wellness Council of the Midlands of South Carolina, was established by the greater Columbia Chamber of Commerce to promote wellness and health-related programs at the worksite, and 35 companies have joined the Council to date. In the view of the Chamber of Commerce, such programs can have a positive impact on the community's economic development activities.

Management firmly believes that the outcome of a strong worksite wellness program is a more productive employee population. Colonial has achieved increased productivity over the past several years, and Time Out For Life is certainly among the factors that contributed to this productivity increase. The company remains committed to the goal of a healthy, happy and high-performance work force.

COMPAQ COMPUTER CORPORATION

Compaq Computer Corporation is a world leader in manufacturing portable business and desk top personal computers. Since its founding in February 1982, the Houston, Texas-based company has set sales and financial records. In 1985, Compaq Computer Corporation became the first company to achieve "Fortune 500" status in less than four years. This phenomenal growth has led to rapid expansion of the Compaq work force and facilities.

People within and outside of Compaq attribute the company's remarkable growth to a number of factors. The company has a strong management team and has built a responsive corporate organization poised to achieve continuing growth. Engineering and marketing savvy stems from listening carefully to customers. Compaq has established standards for performance, quality of design, reliability and superior features that meet computer user needs. A participative management style encourages involvement and innovation.

A strong sense of the value of happy, productive employees permeates the company. Compaq employs more than 7,000 people worldwide, with U.S. and international manufacturing and office facilities totaling more than 2,400,000 square feet. An additional 1,850,000 square feet of office and manufacturing space is under construction.

The care taken to preserve and enhance natural beauty at all of its sites is one of many examples of Compaq's focus on creating a healthful environment for employees. Manufacturing facilities and office buildings are atrium style with natural lighting and tall trees and plants indoors. The Houston site is in a pine woods and features an award-winning natural landscape design with

The material in this contribution appears through the cooperation and permission of Compaq Computer Corporation and Mary Beth McGowen.

picnic areas and a mile-long jogging trail which is being expanded to five miles.

HEALTHPAQ is the Compaq health promotion and fitness program. Its goal is to provide the appropriate information, programs and environment to enable employees and their families to adopt and maintain healthy behaviors, thereby achieving their optimal level of health and well-being. Compaq currently uses many diverse services and activities to achieve wellness. These include programs in recreation, fitness, health education, medical screening, safety, medical benefits, environmental health and communications.

A vast array of recreational activities are provided by the Association of Compaq Employees (ACE). These activities include: softball, basketball, bowling, volleyball, flag football, arts and crafts, Toastmasters, writing, scuba diving, travel tours, golf tournaments and many others. ACE also arranges ticket discounts for various theatre and musical performances. All employees and families are members of this organization. Membership is free. ACE is funded largely by Compaq, with some costs covered by participation fees for certain activities.

Other fitness activities for Houston employees are channeled through a unique association with the YMCA which is adjacent to the Compaq campus. Compaq chose to establish a relationship with the YMCA instead of building its own fitness center for several reasons:

1. The YMCA has a long history of quality staff education and has strong family programs.
2. The YMCA already had a facility and a trained, competent staff.
3. The cost savings of using the YMCA instead of building and operating an on-site facility were significant.

Compaq's agreement with the YMCA calls for the YMCA to discount joining fees in return for a large volume of new members. The YMCA also agreed to expansions and renovations necessary to provide adequate facilities and activities for the increased membership.

Currently 1,400 employees have individual or family memberships at the nearby YMCA with an additional 200 belonging to other YMCAs in the Houston area. Approximately 50 employees and families hold memberships in other regions around the United States. Memberships for Canadian employees are currently being negotiated.

Quarterly corporate donations to the YMCA allow for major renovations and additions to the existing facility including a fitness room with weight training and aerobic equipment overlooking the lake and woods, an aerobics dance room, new locker rooms with saunas and whirlpools and a circuit training room.

A computerized activity tracking system is used. Fitness assessments, reassessments and individualized exercise prescriptions are available to all YMCA members. Basketball, volleyball, racquetball, softball, baseball, soccer, tennis, and golf are offered. Exercise classes include aerobics, swimming, water walking, weight training, etc. Classes are also offered in weight management, prenatal care and back care.

Compaq's health promotion director and several other employees who are active YMCA members serve on the board of advisors. Their input, coupled with the infusion of strongly invested community members, have revitalized the board and allowed improved strategic planning.

Compaq's large health fair in January 1989 launched the expanded health promotion program. Six thousand employees and family members participated in the all-day activities. These included over 90 health, fitness and safety related educational exhibits; 20 different types of screening tests; presentations; exercise demonstrations and healthy refreshments.

Yearly cholesterol and blood pressure screening is offered at all Compaq sites in the U.S. Other on-site programs for Houston employees include: "Healthy Back," first aid, CPR, smoking cessation, "Eating Right," weight management, cancer prevention, and stress and time management.

Each quarter Compaq sponsors programs centered on a new health focus that help employees and family members emphasize a specific area of healthy living. These include: Heart Health, Fitness, Stress Management, Substance Abuse, Cancer Prevention, etc. Each health focus involves specific screenings, lectures, seminars, newsletters and distribution of educational literature for employees and families on each topic.

The recent purchase of 744 wooded acres adjacent to the current headquarters allows for continued expansion of the company. The area surrounding a 38 acre lake is being evaluated for a recreational site with fishing, canoeing, softball, etc. An on-site fitness facility and medical center are also being considered.

While Compaq is a young company with a new health promotion program, its progressive, participative management approach and strong belief in its employees sets the stage for the further development of a highly successful program.

CM ALLIANCE

CM Alliance is a Company of 2,000 employees in Hartford, Connecticut who service our 3,000 field associates throughout the country. Our primary products are Life Insurance, Disability Insurance, and Financial Services. Our Wellness program was started in 1985 as a result of an interest from Employee Advisory Committee and Senior Management's response to rising health care costs. CM has a 5,000 sq. foot Fitness facility in its main home office building and a 900 sq. foot satellite facility in a downtown office. The main facility has a variety of exercise equipment including treadmills, bicycles, rowers, cross-country skier, and weight equipment. Our 1,200 sq. ft. group exercise area is provided for the various level and types of exercise classes including a successful karate class in which a participant can earn various belts.

The Fitness program is open to all employees, full and part time, for a nominal fee collected through bimonthly payroll deductions. Membership entitles a person to a Fitness Assessment including a Health Risk Appraisal, blood chemistry and one-on-one wellness consultation with a qualified Fitness Specialist. This individual health education opportunity is one factor for our very low rate of attrition. Connecticut Mutual's "Vision" is to be "Market Driven, Client Oriented, and Financially Strong." Our Wellness Program accomplishes this "vision" through offering a wide variety of Health & Fitness Programs meeting the needs of a diverse employee population.

The Wellness Program has four full-time staff: One Master's prepared Director, two Fitness Specialists who have a Bachelor's or Master's degree and one clerical support.

The specific Wellness programs currently include:

Nutrition/Weight Loss

CPR

Walking Program

Health Education Topics—Lunchtime lectures

Fitness Program

Smoking Cessation

AIDS Education

Fitness Workshops

Group Exercise Classes

Cancer Education

Blood Pressure Screening

Newsletter

Individual Exercise Program

Several incentive programs are used in the Fitness Center to reward and encourage regular exercise. This "client-oriented" Wellness program addresses the needs of employees who have many different levels of readiness for encouraging healthy habits.

CONOCO

Conoco is a major integrated energy company that focuses primarily on finding and developing crude oil and natural gas reserves, and on manufacturing and selling a wide variety of petroleum-based products. The Company currently operates in approximately 25 countries on six continents and employs approximately 20,000 people worldwide.

Reprinted courtesy of Conoco.

Conoco initiated its employee health and fitness program in 1984 when the Company moved its headquarters from near downtown Houston to its current location in west Houston. The complex that comprises the Company headquarters consists of 16 buildings and houses more than 2,000 employees. The 1.2 million-square-foot facility was designed for convenience, comfort, and productivity.

The comprehensive Conoco Health and Fitness Program emphasizes adoption of wellness behaviors such as an active lifestyle, healthful eating, stress management and low back care. The Program is also an integral part of the Company's concern for a broader range of issues concerning the work culture. These include clean air, pleasant work surroundings, comfortable and functional office furniture and work stations, work/home proximities and supervisor/subordinate relationships.

The strength of the Conoco Health and Fitness Program stems from the commitment and support of executive management and the desire of employees to participate in, and benefit from, a comprehensive corporate wellness program.

ELIGIBILITY

All Houston-based, full-time, salaried employees are eligible to participate in the Health & Fitness Program. In addition, spouses and dependents 14 years or older may use the Fitness Center during special hours.

FACILITIES

Thirteen thousand square feet centrally located in the complex that includes:

Separate men's and women's locker rooms with a total of 1,200 lockers

An exercise room with a variety of aerobic and strength-training equipment

Two classrooms for group exercise and wellness classes
1.35 mile outdoor all-wealther-surface fitness trail

STAFF

Professional Staff
Manager
Three Coordinators
Three Interns
Part-time Nutritionist
Part-time Clinical Social
Worker

Support Staff
One Secretary
Two Receptionists

PROGRAMS

Exercise Classes
Low Impact High Energy
Aerobics
Heavy Hands
Super Circuits
Weekend Workout
Friday Fitness Happy Hour

Hi-Low Aerobics
Weights, Bands & Belles
Pregnancy & You

Wellness Classes
Eating Education
Eating Well in the Working World
Microwave Cooking Series
EAT FOR L.I.F.E.
Cooking for You and Your Kids
Grocery Shopping Tours
Stress Management
Assertiveness Training
Time Management
Effective Communication
Parenting
Women's Issues

Low Back Care
   A Balanced Life, A Balanced Back
   Ergonomic Workplace Assessment & Redesign
Special Promotions
   Attend You Win
   New Games Festival
   Fitness Buddies Inc.
   Test Your Best
   Consistency Club
Other Offerings
   Bike Club
   Running Club
   Brown Bag Sessions
   Eating Well Cafeteria Program
Weekend Workshop
   Meet Your Feet Walking Workshop
   Running Techniques—Gait Analysis
   Bike Repair
   Relaxation Skills
   Infant CPR & Choking
   Breastfeeding
   Infant Care
   Making Good Relationships Better

PROGRAM EVALUATION

Short-Term

1. Examine Changes in Employee Self-Care Behavior/Attitude Toward Health
2. Measure Participant Physiological Changes (after 6 mo. and 1 yr.) of Program Participation
3. Examine Participant Program Satisfaction

---

* Child care is provided for weekend workshops and weekend use of the exercise facility.

Long-Term

1. Following participant trends relative to exercise adherence
2. Measurement of changes in worker productivity and job/ Company satisfaction

Conoco's Company management as well as the management of the Health and Fitness Program feels that a strong evaluation component is critical to the long-term success of a worksite health and fitness program. Prior to implementation of the Health and Fitness Program at Conoco an evaluation plan was put in place to examine both the short-term and long-term effects of the Program. Results of evaluation efforts help make programming more effective, justify the Program to company management and contribute to the worksite wellness profession.

CORNING INCORPORATED

Corning traces its origins to a glass company at Cambridge, Mass., in which Amory Houghton purchased an interest in 1851. Members of the Houghton family have remained active in Corning's business ever since. In 1868, the Houghtons transferred operations to Corning, N.Y., where the Company initially produced thermometer tubing, pharmaceutical glassware, railroad signal glass, and tableware blanks. The company incorporated in 1875 as Corning Glass Works.

Today Corning and its subsidiary companies comprise a worldwide organization with 32 plants, 40 sales and service offices, and approximately 25,000 employees worldwide. Corning is also an investor—with an ownership of 50 percent or less—in 24 affiliated companies in 11 countries. Sales of these equity-based companies, when combined with those of Corning, total some $5 billion annually.

Reprinted courtesy of Corning.

The company competes in four broad business sectors: specialty materials, consumer housewares, laboratory sciences, and telecommunications. Corning produces some 60,000 products; principle trademarks include Corelle, Corning Ware, Pyrex, Steuben and Vycor.

Among Corning's long-held values is "The Individual." The company places great value on its employees, on their individual levels of expertise and their contributions to the company, both singly and collectively. To that end, Corning considers its employee wellness/fitness programs an integral part of the wide range of corporate activities which support that value statement with concrete action.

Corning's PLUS Program is a cluster of practical activities offered in the Corning, N.Y., area (and at certain other Corning locations as well) designed to promote wellness for employees and their families. PLUS includes on-the-job health tests, a comprehensive smoking-cessation program, health-related seminars, and an Employee Guidance and Counseling Program for drug or alcohol abuse, personal finances, marital difficulties or emotional problems.

A popular part of PLUS is Corning's "PLUS Fitness" partnership with the Corning, N.Y., YMCA. This liaison enables the company to offer a broad range of programs which include aerobics, weight training, floor exercises, yoga, proper diet, and care of chronic back problems.

It's one thing to offer fitness programs. It's another matter entirely to create a climate that encourages their use, and encourages employees and their families to stay fit and well. As a first step, Corning provides a one-year full facility YMCA membership to each new employee and his or her family. In addition, Corning pays 50 percent of any employee's PLUS Fitness program fee. If the employee then attends at least 80 percent of the program, the company reimburses the employee's contribution in full. The company also provides fitness program discounts for employees' spouses. (Based on IRS guidelines, the fitness programs are taxable to the employees. The Corning-paid value of the fitness programs is added to the employees' W-2 statements as imputed income at the end of the year.)

Also available in the Corning, N.Y., area, is an employee recreation program which is housed in the Activities Center adjacent to the company's corporate headquarters building.

DOW CHEMICAL COMPANY

The Dow Chemical Company, headquartered in Midland, Michigan, is a diversified manufacturer of more than 1,800 chemicals, plastics, agricultural and consumer products and pharmaceuticals. Founded in 1897 by Herbert H. Dow, Dow is now the sixth largest chemical company in the world in sales with actual 1988 sales of $16.7 billion. Dow and its wholly and partly owned subsidiaries operate plants at 150 locations in 31 countries and maintain 160 sales offices.

In October 1985, Dow instituted a health awareness program for headquarters unit employees. Called "Up With Life," the program has since expanded to include a number of sales offices, manufacturing locations and subsidiaries both inside and outside the U.S. While some basic guidelines have been developed, each location is free to create and tailor the program to best meet its needs. Resources and consulting services are available from the corporate headquarters.

Up With Life is an ongoing, permanent program intended to provide the kind of information and supportive environment that will help employees develop a healthy lifestyle. The program consists of six major components: fitness and exercise, smoking cessation, stress management, nutrition and weight control, cardiovascular fitness, and cancer prevention and early detection.

Up With Life also covers less traditional topics such as child care, care for the elderly and suicide awareness.

All activities are voluntary and draw on a combination of on-site programs and community resources. The number of stimu-

---

Reprinted courtesy of Dow Chemical Company.

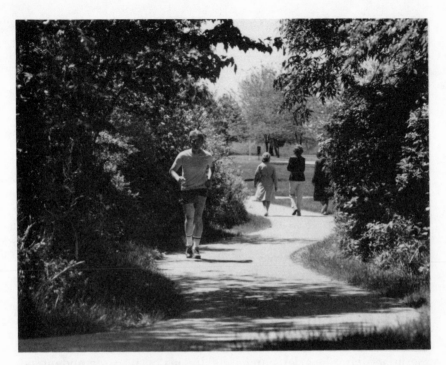

Dow Chemical track in Midland, Michigan.

lating, interesting programs is intended to make employees realize that maintaining a healthy lifestyle is part of the fun of living.

FITNESS AND EXERCISE

While sit-ups, push-ups and pull-ups are traditional forms of fitness, Up With Life utilizes programs like aerobics and belly-shapers which are a bit more fun. These, along with a wide variety of other exercise options, help employees reduce stress and weight, lower their risk of heart attack, raise energy levels and improve self-esteem.

The programs are designed to accommodate various levels of motivation and expertise from novice on up.

At Dow's headquarters, employees enjoy working out in Up With Life's functional in-house exercise facilities or running the

1.5-mile outdoor track. In Sarnia, Ontario, the location of Dow Canada's headquarters, exercise facilities are also available for employees' use. Other Dow locations, which may not have exercise facilities on site, have opted to rent space at community centers, encourage walking or running groups and utilize a variety of other creative methods to encourage fitness.

SMOKING CESSATION

Health risks associated with smoking are formidable and real. Up With Life offers a variety of methods that focus on learning new behavior. Also available are general clinics, self-help workbooks, and seminars on smoking and related topics.

STRESS MANAGEMENT

At one time or another, most people are subject to high stress levels. Stress—and the accompanying depression, negative feelings and vulnerability to disease and accidents—can sap one's strength and take the joy out of living.

Through Up With Life, employees are presented with insights and tools to help manage stress. Proper stress management can help maintain self-confidence, peace of mind, motivation and a productive, positive attitude.

NUTRITION AND WEIGHT CONTROL

Proper nutrition and weight control can result in better health and reduced risk of disease. More energy, higher self-esteem and a better outlook are other benefits.

Up With Life offers a variety of programs to address a number of dietary issues, including weight control, the nutritional value of fast foods, computerized diet assessment, and dietary pitfalls—such as the problems with excess sodium intake.

CARDIOVASCULAR FITNESS

In addition to fitness and exercise programs, Up With Life specialists perform regular blood pressure screening and address a number of topics specifically designed to help employees keep their hearts healthy and pumping more efficiently.

UP WITH LIFE IS FOR EVERYONE

Research studies show that people who live a healthy lifestyle are happier and live longer. Indications are that these people are also more dependable employees. Their outlook is better, enthusiasm is higher, absenteeism due to minor illness is minimized and time off due to major medical causes is reduced.

Employee participation has been overwhelmingly enthusiastic since the Up With Life program's inception in 1985. The program teaches employees to change their lifestyle—a little at a time. Through a series of small changes, employees can improve not only the quality, but also the quantity of their days.

DU PONT

The Du Pont Company began offering employees participation in a comprehensive health promotion program in June 1984. Designed to familiarize workers with the relationship of good health habits and good health, the program was offered to 89,000 people at 85 sites in the first five years.

In 1981, Du Pont laid the groundwork by hiring Robert L. Bertera, who recently had earned his doctor of public health degree from Johns Hopkins University in Baltimore. He was named manager of health promotion programs and based at company headquarters in Wilmington, Del.

For a year after joining Du Pont, Bertera researched other

Reprinted courtesy of Du Pont Co. and R. B. Young and R. L. Bertera.

corporate wellness efforts, then in their infancy. He sifted through massive amounts of health data and studies compiled by Du Pont over the years. He also kept up to date on the latest findings on the relationship of lifestyle and health and began to recruit and train a group of health professionals.

During the preliminary phase, Bertera determined that a workable plan would have to be voluntary and confidential. Otherwise, the company was unlikely to get the employee participation necessary for meaningful, long-term change.

Bertera also realized that an effective program needed to be comprehensive; that is, not limited to a single health risk factor such as smoking or fitness. Early on, he identified six controllable health factors thought to be closely linked with lifestyle: stress management, smoking cessation, weight and lipid control, blood pressure control, fitness, and a healthy back. Dental care was added to the list later.

At Bertera's recommendation, Du Pont decided to test an innovative, multi-faceted program involving leadership training, initial health-risk assessments, and lifestyle-changing activities. The aim was to decrease health-care costs by improving employee health.

"The beauty of the wellness program at Du Pont is that it's good for the company and it's good for employees," Bertera says. "It serves a very important function at this company."

As its first test, Du Pont launched a pilot program at its plant in Memphis, Tenn., in 1981. After initial promotion, 75 percent of the labor force turned out to complete an easy-to-read, 10-minute, 38-question health risk survey about their health status, personal habits, and lifestyles.

The forms were then analyzed on computers. Within a month, each person received an individualized, confidential assessment of the health risks involved in his or her lifestyle.

The employees then were invited to attend educational programs on the seven health priorities. Most initial sessions featured speeches, videotapes, slide shows, audio tapes, and participatory puzzles and quizzes.

Motivated by the introductory presentations, many employees began a series of wellness-oriented group activities sponsored in the workplace. Others chose self-help kits, books, or tapes to make health improvements on their own. T-shirts, mugs, and similar incentives were offered to promote weight-loss contests, blood pressure screenings, and other activities on and off the job.

Within a short period, Du Pont verified a significant drop in disability wages and other health costs at the pilot program in Memphis. The savings was attributed to the workplace wellness program.

And the change has continued. During a recent six-year period, the Tennessee plant experienced a 47.5 decrease in lost workdays. Since the program began, management has spent about $119,000 less each year on disability wages for the overall plant, representing a return of more than $2 on every $1 invested by the company.

Encouraged by results of the pilot program, Du Pont decided in 1984 to offer an expanded version to 120 locations companywide. It set up three core elements for sites wishing to offer the program: coordinator training, health-risk assessment, and health promotion activities.

The first component involves a three-day workshop for site leaders, medical personnel, and health promotion activity committee members. Believing in local autonomy, Du Pont encourages site coordinators to customize offerings to their particular needs.

The second step is completion of the health-risk assessment. Like their Memphis predecessors, employees later receive specific suggestions and literature about problem areas such as smoking.

The third core element is the activities phase. Although the company in some cases has constructed on-site walking and jogging trails, outfitted equipment rooms, and sponsored aerobic classes, it relies on outside agencies such as the YWCA for most facilities and instructors.

To maintain continued enthusiasm for wellness, Du Pont publishes and distributes a quarterly newsletter with articles about activities at various sites. It also stages an annual program review conference for site wellness coordinators and committee members.

Like Memphis, 11 other sites are showing substantial reductions in disability wage costs. Since launching the program, they also have experienced an average return of more than $2 for every $1 invested.

According to Burford W. Culpepper, M.D., Director of Du Pont's Medical Division, the effort has been a resounding success.

"Our wellness program has been received with tremendous enthusiasm, " Dr. Culpepper says. "It recognizes increased employee interest in health improvement and is in keeping with a consensus of medical opinion that shows it is more effective to place emphasis on prevention of illness through practice of good health habits than to rely solely on routine periodic physical examinations."

Among satisfied participants are Paul Kugelman, manufacturing technical manager for "Orlon" in Wilmington, and Selina Vincent, a secretary at the Chambers Works plant in Deepwater, N.J. Through the Du Pont wellness program, Kugelman became involved in a regular fitness regimen while Vincent got control of her weight.

Kugelman credits the program with giving him needed incentive to get fit. Encouragement from other Du Pont employees, he claims, was crucial to his success.

"I try to exercise three or four times a week, and I've been doing that pretty consistently for the last several years," he says. "What I find is that the program helps me with self-discipline, because it's really tough to do it by yourself."

Similarly, Vincent praises the program for motivating her to shed extra pounds. Dieting with a group of other women at her plant she relies on group support for emotional reinforcement.

"We have all kinds of things in our lunchroom hanging on the walls that tell us calories and nutritional items, " Vincent says. "We have books there, and we have lunch together, which helps, because we're always checking one another and seeing what we're eating or what new thing we could eat that's lower in fat or calories.

"We really, really support one another, which is the best part of the program, " Vincent says. "You're not doing it alone. You don't have anyone tempting you. We eat lunch together so if we're all eating diet foods, there's no temptation."

Where do Du Pont's health and wellness efforts go from here? According to Bertera, the program will continue to respond to economic and social changes affecting the company.

Already in the works are efforts to involve more families, who account for two-thirds of insurance costs. The health promotion staff is brainstorming ways to bolster appeal to spouses, family members, sales and field personnel, and pensioners.

In addition, the company plans to add more health topics to the original seven. Among those being developed is AIDS education.

Bertera, whose budget jumped to $1.2 million from $60,000 in the first five years of the program, thinks wellness efforts will be a permanent fixture on the corporate scene. He dismisses any notion that interest in health and fitness may be just a short-term fad.

"I believe there has been a fundamental change in the last 15 or 20 years in our understanding of the role that lifestyle plays in how we feel, how long we live, and our quality of life," Bertera says. "Certainly, over time there will be changes and new additions to information we have in areas such as fitness an nutrition. But I just can't imagine a return to the days when we virtually ignored lifestyle factors."

THE EASTMAN KODAK COMPANY

Kodak was founded in 1880 by George Eastman, who simplified photography and built a mass market for film and cameras. More than 100 years later, Kodak remains the world's premier imaging company.

With sales in excess of $17 billion, Kodak ranked 18th on the most recent list of the Fortune 500 companies. Headquartered in Rochester, N.Y., it employs approximately 145,000 people in more than 150 countries.

Kodak films and cameras are household items for most consumers. Its diagnostic imaging products are equally familiar to physicians, and its motion picture film stock is the preferred choice of most Hollywood cinematographers.

The company also is a major, multi-billion-dollar supplier of commercial and information imaging systems for today's electronic office. In recent years, the company has added a wide range of bi-products and pharmaceuticals for the burgeoning life sciences industry. Kodak's latest expansion in this direction was the acquisition of Sterling Drug Inc., which added Bayer aspirin and Lysol disinfectant to the Kodak family of products.

Kodak also is underwriting a variety of small venture groups both within and outside the company as an investment in future chemical, electronic and optical technologies.

Kodak's tradition of concern for the health of its employees dates back at least to 1914, when the company medical department began publishing monthly health bulletins with titles such as "Rupture," "Rest & Sleep," and "Germs."

That same year, the company began sponsoring employee recreation programs which have grown steadily ever since. Kodak also was in the vanguard of companies that developed active programs in the 1940s to combat industrial alcoholism.

MANAGEMENT PHILOSOPHY

The main thrust of Kodak's fitness effort is fueled by the company's "Life Enhancement Plan." Conceived by Kodak Medical Director, Dr. James Mitchell, it encompasses many programs designed to spur employees to take responsibility for their own physical and mental well-being.

Kodak advances this concept by encouraging employees to avail themselves of corporate resources that promote health and enhance the quality of life. These resources fall into three categories: (a) health & safety education, (b) health appraisals, and (c) fitness.

The company administers many of its Life Enhancement programs through Occupational Health & Safety Teams, each consisting of a Kodak physician, at least one registered nurse plus support from Safety and Administrative Services. About 20 of these teams serve Kodak employees in Rochester, revolving among internal client organizations to provide health services.

HEALTH & SAFETY EDUCATION

Kodak offers a broad array of educational programs about health issues including nutrition, weight reduction, substance abuse, smoking cessation, stress management and breast cancer detection. Some of these are administered by the Occupational Health & Safety Teams; others are run by outside agencies retained to conduct seminars at Kodak sites during the noon hour or after work.

The stress management program, for example, is run by the American Red Cross for Kodak employees and their families at each of the company's three major employment centers in Rochester.

HEALTH APPRAISAL

The flagship program under this component of the Life Enhancement Plan is Cardiovascular Risk Control (CVRC). A three-stage program administered by Occupational Health & Safety Teams, it seeks to: (a) identify persons at high risk of developing coronary disease, (b) arrange for community physicians to treat them, and (c) monitor employees' compliance with plans prescribed by their doctors. Internal communications urge employees to schedule risk evaluations. For example, a 12-minute video entitled "Cholesterol Control" is shown continuously during lunch time in Kodak cafeterias.

FITNESS

Aerobics classes are taught at lunch time and after hours by professional instructors who conduct workouts on the premises at Kodak's main employment centers. The company subsidizes costs so that employees pay only a nominal fee.

A fitness program for employees is administered by the Recreation Department with consultation and support from Occupational Health & Safety Teams.

Morale-building incentives for participation in these programs include lettered caps and t-shirts that advertise "personal best" performances.

Kodak also sponsors one of the largest intramural team sports programs in corporate America. League schedules show 120 basketball teams, 130 volleyball teams, 220 softball teams and 50 soccer teams. Kodak-subsidized tournaments include bowling, golf, tennis and squash invitationals.

Company-owned and operated facilities include three full-court gymnasiums, 17 softball fields, 10 lighted tennis courts, four soccer fields, and several squash courts.

The Medical Department's Sports Injury Reduction Committee promotes safe practices in sports and prescribes "warm-up" and "cool-down" exercise regimens for all sports. Since the panel's formation in 1984, athletic injuries in Kodak-sponsored contests have been reduced by about 40 percent, and lost work days due to such injuries have been cut by more than 60 percent.

EMPLOYEE ASSISTANCE PROGRAM

Because mental and physical fitness can be affected by personal problems, Kodak administers a voluntary confidential Employee Assistance Program that provides short-term counseling, assessment, referral and follow-up for employees and their families. Organized in 1985, the free service is an outgrowth of Kodak's industrial alcoholism program, and about 20 percent of the current caseload involves substance abuse. Another 30 percent consists of employees seeking professional, legal or financial assistance. Family, marital and emotional problems account for the remaining 50 percent.

SELF-CARE CENTERS

Among the most visible symbols of Kodak's emphasis on personal responsibility are the medical department's Self-Care Centers. These are small unstaffed stations in high-traffic areas where employees can weigh themselves, check their blood pressure and get aspirin or other over-the-counter medicines from a vending machine. The centers encourage self-reliance and help free Kodak medical personnel to treat more seriously ill employees.

THE FUTURE

Currently, about 20 percent of Kodak's Rochester-based workforce participates in some form of company-sponsored fitness/wellness program. With the growth of services offered under the Life Enhancement umbrella, Kodak expects to increase that figure to 60 percent within five years.

LIFEKEY®* ELECTRONIC DATA SYSTEMS

Electronic Data Systems Corporation (EDS) is a people-oriented information services company owned by General Motors. EDS is one of the largest, most respected data processing companies in the world. More than 6,000 employees work at the corporate headquarters in Dallas, and 46,000 more are located at sites nationally and internationally.

In 1984, the Health and Fitness Division was formed, which subsequently created the Lifekey® wellness program to meet several goals:

- To create an awareness of potential health risks.
- To advise individuals at increased health risk to actively seek medical consultation for primary care.
- To encourage personal responsibility for health and fitness.
- To provide accurate, nonbiased information pertaining to health and fitness.
- To provide convenient, low-cost wellness programs

Reprinted courtesy of Electronic Data Systems Corporation.

*Lifekey is a registered trademark of Electronic Data Systems Corporation.

and activities that support voluntary lifestyle changes toward optimal health.

Full-time health promotion specialists work out of three regional sites (each run by an area manager). In addition, to reach remote sites, more than 700 employee volunteers serve as Health and Fitness coordinators. They form the communication link between the division and employees by distributing information, planning programs, and at sites not having a fitness facility, are encouraged to arrange health club discounts.

The Lifekey® program believes motivation is the key to lifestyle change. Since 1984, three needs analyses of its population have been conducted. Each one illustrated that EDS employees are well aware of what they should be doing to get and stay healthy. What they lack is the appropriate motivational tools to make changes in their lives.

HEARTCHEK

HeartChek is a screening program that Lifekey® instituted to test employee's blood cholesterol, blood pressure, body fat composition, and cardiac risk (through a questionnaire). Following the screening, a follow-up class is presented during which participants receive their results and learn ways to reduce their cardiac risk.

In 1989, Lifekey® began targeting specific accounts with the HeartChek programs. Once employees are screened, results are tabulated and an aggregate report is presented to that account's manager, along with specific recommendations to reduce risk factors in that population. Recommendations may include exercise programs, cholesterol education, stress management, and smoking cessation referrals.

FITNESS

Lifekey® encourages physical activity in ways that are geared toward particular employee groups. In some instances, group competition is the best motivator; in other cases, individual awards provide the incentive to begin and maintain an exercise program.

Fitness classes and clinics provide expert instruction on subjects such as general conditioning, fitness for women, and exercise safety. A software program is also available to help monitor daily exercise and nutrition habits.

To promote aerobic fitness, an Activity Log is accessible to everyone at EDS. This mainframe computer-based system allows users to record their participation in various aerobic activities and receive points that reflect the level of aerobic benefit, as well as the caloric expenditure for each activity.

The Log is not only a tool for maintaining aerobic fitness, but also for developing long-range fitness goals. Periodic competitions among Log users provide fun incentives for continuing effective aerobic exercise programs.

NUTRITION

Being well includes eating well, and Lifekey® helps employees understand the impact of nutrition on wellness in the following ways:

- Classes and seminars presented by registered dietitians emphasize the value of good nutrition to overall health.
- The "Healthy Heart" menu, a selection of foods low in fat, cholesterol and sodium, is available in company eating areas.
- Weight loss competitions and incentive programs help motivate employees to shed excess pounds.
- A computer-based instruction program is available to all employees to enhance their knowledge of nutrition and provide guidelines for healthy eating. This program is also available in an audiotape version.
- A comprehensive nutritional evaluation, recommendations for improved eating habits, and personalized menu plans are available through the Health Assessment Program.

HEALTH ASSESSMENT PROGRAM

The Health Assessment program is a vital part of Lifekey®. Through intensive testing, professional evaluation and follow-up, employees learn their health-risk status and are given information to maintain or improve their current health.

The comprehensive Health Assessment involves several aspects:

- Present health/risk status is assessed to identify the likelihood of disease, disability or premature death.
- Current nutritional practices are evaluated.
- A variety of tests are performed, including a blood chemistry analysis, an EKG-monitored submaximal stress test, vital lung capacity, body fat composition, pulmonary function, flexibility and muscular strength.
- Specific lifestyle changes necessary for optimal health are identified and defined.

Based upon these findings, registered dietitians and exercise physiologists provide individual menu planning and exercise recommendations. The staff works directly with each participant to develop a practical plan for reducing risks and improving their potential for good health.

SUMMARY

Lifekey's success at EDS is measurable not only in interest and participation, but also through scientific surveys conducted periodically among employees. For example, between 1984 and 1988 the program documented decreases in the number of employees who smoke and in absenteeism, while increases were observed for variables such as seat-belt usage and the number of employees who are eating healthier.

For more information about the Lifekey program, please contact Electronic Data Systems, 5400 Legacy Drive, Plano, Texas 75024 or call (214) 661-6000.

FORD MOTOR COMPANY

Ford Motor Company is a worldwide leader in automotive and automotive-related products and services as well as in newer industries such as aerospace, communications, and financial services. While there are more than 350,000 Ford Motor Company employees throughout the world, the following description of employee assistance and health promotion services applies only to approximately 155,000 hourly and salaried men and women working in the United States and employed by the parent company and certain major subsidiaries.

A CHANGING CORPORATE CULTURE

To fully understand employee assistance and health promotion services at Ford, they should be viewed in the context of a changing corporate culture.

During the early 1980s an intentional process of corporate transformation was initiated. The broad direction for this transformation is best described in Ford Motor Company's "Mission, Values and Guiding Principles." In listing the Company's core values—people, products and profits—it states: "Our people are the source of our strength. They provide our corporate intelligence and determine our reputation and vitality. Involvement and teamwork are our core human values."

With people and teamwork as central values, this cultural transformation has resulted in an increasing emphasis upon the development of our human resources and their contribution to the success of the business.

HUMAN RESOURCES

A variety of approaches have been employed to provide opportunities to increase the capacity, capability and commitment of Ford people. These approaches include opportunities for more partici-

Reprinted courtesy of Ford Motor Company.

pation and involvement in the work process. They also include more technical training and job skills development than ever before, along with opportunities for continuing personal and career education and development, and training in health and safety practices at work.

For the approximately 105,000 UAW-represented Ford employees in the U.S., many of these approaches are joint efforts between Ford and the UAW. At every level, Company and Union representatives work together to assure that the joint activities are high quality and meet the needs of hourly employees.

EMPLOYEE ASSISTANCE AND HEALTH PROMOTION

Included in these efforts to focus on the importance of our people are new directions and emphasis on employee assistance and health promotion services.

Employee assistance and health promotion services for UAW-represented employees are delivered through the UAW-Ford Employee Assistance Plan (EAP). Ford and the UAW negotiated the UAW-Ford EAP as part of the 1984 Collective Bargaining Agreement. The comparable program for salaried employees is called Total Health. Each of these programs is designed to help employees to resolve existing personal and health problems (employee assistance) and to avoid potential problems through lifestyle modification (health promotion).

Leadership for the UAW-Ford EAP is provided by a national committee which is composed of an equal number of representatives from the Company and the Union.

At each major plant, a full-time Union EAP Representative has been selected from the local union to serve the UAW-Ford EAP. Smaller locations have a part-time Union EAP Representative. Every location also has a part-time Company representative serving the UAW-Ford EAP. Ongoing training is provided for both Company and Union selected UAW-Ford EAP Representatives. In addition to these representatives, local UAW-Ford EAP Committees have also been established at every plant and parts distribution center. Together the local committees and representatives are responsible for local program planning, promotion, training, delivery and monitoring of services for UAW-represented employees.

The Total Health program, which provides employee assistance and health promotion services for salaried employees, has a national level committee of management representatives from major Company components similar to the UAW-Ford EAP. It is administered at the national and division level by Total Health Coordinators. Most locations have a part-time local Total Health Representative, and many locations have local Total Health Committees. Whenever practical and appropriate, employee assistance and health promotion activities are delivered to hourly and salaried employees in tandem to assure uniformity of service.

PROGRAM SERVICES

All direct professional services for both the UAW-Ford EAP and Total Health are delivered by contract providers. Professional employee assistance counseling goes beyond the traditional employee assistance focus and provides confidential assistance to employees and their families for any personal, health or lifestyle concern. Professional employee assistance services are delivered by independent employee assistance service providers who are not associated with treatment facilities. In addition to employee assistance counseling for employees and family members, both the UAW-Ford EAP and Total Health also include consultation for supervisors regarding employees who are experiencing declines in performance or conduct which may be associated with a personal problem.

Health promotion activities include health risk appraisal, hypertension and cholesterol screening and follow-up, smoking cessation, and education in nutrition, exercise, and stress management. The on-site health risk appraisal and hypertension and cholesterol screening for hourly and salaried employees at plants and parts distribution centers were specially designed for use in manufacturing facilities.

Several weeks after the appraisal and screening, each participant receives a personal and confidential health assessment report. This report advises the participant on ways in which they can enhance their well-being, and indicates specific problem resolution and lifestyle modification activities available through the UAW-Ford EAP or Total Health.

Cholesterol screening is completed on-site through the use of the dry-chemistry blood analysis method. Participants who have cholesterol and/or blood pressure readings in the moderate or high range are invited to participate in follow-up screening after six, twelve and eighteen months. With the employee's permission, results of the screening are shared with the employee's personal physician. Individual results of health risk appraisal and screening activities, as with all other health promotion and employee assistance activities, are strictly confidential.

Exercise education activities are delivered through three different options: exercise information, exercise education by demonstration, and exercise classes. Neither the UAW-Ford EAP nor Total Health provides for the development of on-site exercise facilities or membership in health clubs. The purpose of exercise education is to encourage exercise through increased awareness and education, but not to provide unlimited continuing support of individual exercise programs.

Nutrition education activities are also available through three different options: general nutrition, weight management, and heart healthy education. The heart healthy education option is specifically targeted to assist participants with respect to cardiovascular risk.

Smoking cessation classes also are offered, but they are not a "one shot" intervention. Rather, they extend over a period of time, have as their basis education and a planned sequence of behavior modification, and include a minimum of three "maintenance" sessions after completion of the intervention or "stop smoking" phase of the program.

Stress management activities for hourly and salaried employees at plants and parts distribution centers normally are delivered by the local employee assistance counseling service following an approved format. The goal of stress management education is to help the employee recognize sources and symptoms of their stress, and to create a personal action plan which encourages them to utilize employee assistance, health promotion and other educational activities available to them.

CREATING A HEALTHY COMPANY

Ford Motor Company recognizes that individual efforts to resolve personal problems and to enhance personal health and lifestyle must be supported by a healthy environment at work. Joint Company- and Union-sponsored health and safety training and research, ergonomic studies, participative management and employee involvement activities, and education and training opportunities all contribute to creating a healthy workplace.

FUTURE ACTIVITIES

The future success of these activities will depend upon continued leadership and support from the top levels of both the Company and the UAW, and on UAW-Ford EAP and Total Health Representatives and Committees at the local level continuing to develop and customize employee assistance and health promotion activities to meet the needs of employees and family members. Ford recognizes that "people are the source of our strength," and Ford, working jointly with the UAW, is committed to cultivating this strength through employee assistance and health promotion activities.

GANNETT

Gannett is a nationwide information company that publishes 85 daily newspapers, including USA TODAY, 35 non-daily newspapers and USA WEEKEND, a newspaper magazine. It also operates 10 television stations and 16 radio stations and owns the largest outdoor advertising company in North America. Gannett is headquartered in Arlington, Virginia.

Gannett also has marketing, television news and programming production, research satellite information systems and a national group of commercial printing facilities. Gannett has operations in 41 states, the District of Columbia, Guam, the Virgin Islands, Canada, Great Britain, Hong Kong, Singapore and Switzerland.

Health/works, the Gannett health and fitness center, is conveniently located between the twin towers of the Gannett & USA TODAY headquarters in Arlington, Virginia. Employees have easy access to the 20,000-square-foot facility which includes a medical area, health education classroom, health resource area, juice bar, exercise classroom and the main exercise area. A running track encloses the main exercise area which features Keiser series 300 pneumatic resistance equipment, biocycles, treadmills, rowing ergometers, Stairmasters and cross-country ski machines.

Two well-known independent groups have been contracted to provide the services for health/works. Fitness Systems, which provides consulting management and facility design expertise in fitness and health education programs to businesses nationwide, manages the facility and supervises the health and fitness programs. Options & Choices, which provides a broad range of medical prevention and consultative services, developed and is providing medical and prevention services. Fitness Systems provides Gannett with professional and support staff ensuring quality by identifying individuals well-trained in the areas of exercise physiology, health education and recreation, combined with enthusiastic personalities. Options and Choices staffs the Medical Department with two Master's-level Nurse Clinicians. A medical doctor is on site two days per week.

The health/works program has been tailored specifically to the needs of Gannett and USA TODAY employees. A health/works committee consisting of Gannett and USA TODAY employees was developed to guide in the initial planning of the facility and currently serves as an important link to the employee population. All 1,400 headquarters and USA TODAY staff are eligible to join health/works. Employees from any of Gannett's 147 nationwide operating units may also use the facility during their visits to Arlington.

Membership in health/works is voluntary. All members are given a preliminary health-fitness evaluation, one-on-one with an exercise physiologist followed by a personal fitness profile and exercise prescription and an orientation to the facility. Members pay a one-time enrollment fee of $25.00 and $8.00 per month in dues. In addition to the wide variety of cardiovascular and strength training equipment, health/works members also enjoy a putting green and golf driving range. All Gannett and USA TODAY employees may participate in the health education classes, programs and talks, use the medical department services and enjoy the juice bar/health education resource area, regardless of whether or not they choose to join health/works.

The health/works philosophy follows a three-step approach recognizing the varying needs of the employees we serve. For each intervention, employees may select from self-help resources, an individualized program, or a structured, organized class. All resources are carefully screened and selected by the health/works staff. Although many of our programs are taught by health/works staff, outside vendors are also brought in to provide the utmost in quality to our employees.

Our exercise class schedule, featuring aerobics, conditioning, stretching, yoga, karate, jazz and ballroom dance, provides variety and varying degrees of intensity for all fitness levels. Twenty-five classes per week are offered.

A key ingredient to the success of any program is visible, high-level support. Gannett's senior management actively participate in the programming at health/works, in addition to lending a great deal of support, which contributes to the success of the program. Creative programming, effective leadership and the other criteria for success indicated by the President's Council are all aspects of the facility and program at Gannett.

There is something for everyone at health/works. The diverse programs provide an opportunity for all Gannett/USA TODAY employees to strive for better health.

GENERAL MILLS

General Mills has been a major food manufacturer for the past 59 years. Today, General Mills has approximately 74,000 employees. The company consists of two main parts. The Consumer Foods Group produces the familiar product lines such as Gold Medal Flour, Betty Crocker products, Big G cereals, Yoplait yogurt, and Gorton's seafoods. The Restaurant group operates international restaurant chains such as Red Lobster, York's and The Olive Garden.

The health promotion programs are managed by the Department of Health and Human Services, which is involved in medical services, occupational health and safety, recreation/fitness and special services. General Mills has been involved in health promotion for several years. The objective of health promotion at General Mills is to educate the employee through several formats including publications, seminars, formal classes and actual participation in healthy lifestyles. Most health education programs are developed at the Minneapolis headquarters and later introduced at other General Mills locations.

General Mills offers a variety of health promotion classes on a continuing basis at their main offices in Minneapolis. Fitness and aerobic classes are held after work daily. These classes are led by qualified fitness instructors who tailor exercise sessions to the abilities of the participants. All participants are screened before entering the fitness classes. There are fitness facilities with a variety of equipment at several General Mills locations. Smoking cessation classes are offered quarterly. This eight-session class meets twice a week and includes sections on: reasons why people smoke, stress management, mastering the obstacles of quitting, good nutrition, exercise and enjoying life after tobacco. General Mills has also been involved in organizing and participating in Minnesota D-Day (the Great American Smoke-Out) for several

Reprinted courtesy of General Mills.

years. In September 1987, the Minneapolis General Offices became a smoke-free workplace. The weight loss classes are conducted on-site by the Weight Watchers at Work Program. Nutrition information is also available through the General Mills Nutrition Department. The hypertension program is conducted through medical screening of employees with high blood pressure and making follow-up and maintenance data available to the employees' private physicians. Employees are also offered in-house counseling and classes in stress management and chemical dependency. Other classes available to General Mills employees include cardiopulmonary resuscitation (CPR), first aid and breast self-examination.

The General Mills TriHealthalon® program was developed five years ago to expand the health promotion programs to employees who did not have access to the formal education classes offered at the corporate headquarters. The title TriHealthalon® comes from the World Health Organization's definition of good health, which is comprised of physical, mental and social well-being. Participants in this voluntary program must complete a Lifestyle Appraisal. The appraisal is computer-analyzed and returned to the participants as a goal-setting mechanism, which recommends how the participants can improve their health by improving their lifestyle. The results of the Lifestyle Appraisal are kept strictly confidential. The program is then self-directed with the participants using the TriHealthalon® handbook as a guide to a healthy lifestyle. The participants report their healthy lifestyle achievements quarterly with an Activity Record Sheet. There are many options to take in developing a healthy lifestyle and the participants are given credit whether they are beginning in a healthy lifestyle program or have been active in their own health and well-being for a long time. Individuals who have achieved their healthy lifestyle goals receive an incentive award for a job well done. Team awards are also available.

The TriHealthalon® has been quite successful. After two years, improvements in the following lifestyle risk factors have been seen in the participant population: smoking has decreased by 5%, the number of people who use their safety belts has increased by 37%, and there has been a 23% increase in the number of people who exercise three times a week. Absenteeism is also significantly less in the participant groups compared to individuals in the same division who did not participate in the TriHealthalon®.

Health promotion at General Mills utilizes a variety of programs. These programs are designed to make employees more aware of health risks and alternate lifestyle choices. The ultimate goal of these programs is to present information in such a way that the employee takes responsibility to develop and maintain a health lifestyle.

GENERAL MOTORS

General Motors has 210 operations in 30 states and 125 cities in the United States. Of these, 32 are engaged in the final assembly of GM cars and trucks; 14 are Service Parts Operations responsible for distribution or warehousing; 14 are associated with Electronic Data Systems Corporation as a large information processing center; 22 major plants, offices and research facilities relate to the operations of Hughes Aircraft Company; and the remainder are involved primarily in the manufacture of automotive components and power products.

In addition the Corporation has 18 plants in Canada and assembly, manufacturing, distribution or warehousing operations in 33 other countries including equity interests in associated companies which conduct assembly, manufacturing or distribution operations in the U.S. and overseas countries.

The principal operations in the U.S. and Canada are contained in three vehicle groups which include engineering, manufacturing and assembly: Buick-Oldsmobile-Cadillac; Chevrolet-Pontiac-GM of Canada; and Truck and Bus Group.

As of December 1987, our total worldwide employment (exclusive of GM Hughes Electronics Corporation, EDS Corporation and GMAC) was 702,000. Of that total, there are 366,000 hourly employees and 114,000 salaried employees in the U.S. alone.

Reprinted courtesy of General Motors.

At General Motors health promotion is part of our basic operating philosophy. In the United States and Canada, GM employs approximately 1,000 full-time medical staff—physicans, nurses, x-ray technicians, and physicians' assistants. In 1986, approximately six million patient services were provided to GM employees. In addition to complete medical exams for a large number of employees, these services also included medical intervention (and counselling) of considerable scope.

At GM, company-wide programs have been in effect for many years:

Employee Assistance Program (EAP)	1972
Hypertension Screening	1979

The Employee Assistance Program provided treatment for 14,164 employees in 1987. In a joint union-management effort, the EAP offers counselling as well as in-patient and out-patient treatment for GM employees. Our health insurance coverage also provides assistance for dependents as well as GM retirees.

The Hypertension Screening Program was developed with the National Heart, Lung and Blood Institute (NHLBI) and the University of Michigan Institute of Labor and Industrial Relations. Through 1987 the total number of employees screened (including rescreens and medical treatment interventions) has reached 325,000 individuals. Results show that 18 percent of employees had hypertension and one-third were unaware of their condition.

At all GM plants and offices other health promotion interventions include:

Smoking Cessation (in 1985 GM introduced its first policy on smoking and revised it in 1987).

CPR Training

Cancer Screening

Stress Management

Cholesterol Screening

Diabetes Screening

Nutrition Counselling

Aerobics and Exercise Classes

Back Care

First Aid

Health Education

In 1985, a jointly funded research project was started to evaluate various types of wellness interventions at four GM plants in the Detroit area. The results will be published in 1989 by the NHLBI and the University of Michigan.

In 1987, General Motors and the UAW commenced an AIDS Awareness Education Program for all employees and retirees.

Also in 1987, a joint union/management task force was established to design a corporate-wide health promotion program with uniform guidelines for implementation. This joint task force and the future promotional program will be promoted in whole or part by joint union/management health and safety funds.

GENERAL MOTORS CORPORATION

Worksite Smoking Policy

It is now clear that disease risk due to inhalation of tobacco smoke is not solely limited to the individual who is smoking, but can also extend to those individuals who inhale tobacco smoke in room air.
C. Everet Koop, M.D.
United States Surgeon General

PURPOSE

General Motors Corporation recognizes an individual's *right to decide* personal smoking behavior. It is the policy of General Motors, however, to make all reasonable efforts to protect nonsmokers from involuntary exposure to environmental tobacco smoke while in company facilities.

ASSISTANCE

The American Cancer Society indicates the vast majority of smokers would be interested in reducing or quitting smoking if opportunities were made available. Local units will assist in finding and/or implementing cessation programs for GM employees who are interested in becoming nonsmokers.

AREAS WHERE SMOKING IS PERMITTED

Smoking will be permitted except as noted below. Where the preferences of smokers and nonsmokers conflict, local units of General Motors will seek a reasonable resolution consistent with the company's traditional respect for the individual. When seeking resolution, local units should consider individual sensitivities to tobacco smoke and seek to use existing physical barriers whenever possible.

AREAS WHERE SMOKING IS RESTRICTED

All employee cafeterias will provide for both "Smoking" and "No Smoking" areas.

AREAS WHERE SMOKING IS PROHIBITED

Smoking will not be permitted in any area in which a potential safety hazard exists. In addition, to protect nonsmokers, smoking is not permitted in conference rooms, classrooms, elevators, hallways, stairwells, lobbies, waiting rooms, copier rooms, auditoriums, reception areas, company vehicles when transporting both smokers and nonsmokers, and other areas as local units may designate.

IMPLEMENTATION

This policy will become effective September 1, 1987. Educational information and smoking cessation opportunities will be made available for all employees. Local units are encouraged to form a committee of employees consisting of both smokers and non-smokers alike which will accept the responsibility of overseeing the implementation of this smoking policy.

The success of this policy will depend upon the thoughtfulness, consideration, and cooperation of all employees and does not supersede provisions of collective bargaining agreements or posted shop rules and established guidelines for employee conduct.

GENERAL MOTORS POLICY ON SMOKING

While it is not the intent of General Motors to take issue with the smoking preferences of individuals, smoking in the work place is a matter of continuing concern to many employees. Accordingly, General Motors has developed the following policy:

It is the policy of General Motors to respect the preferences of both the non-smoker and the smoker in Company buildings and facilities.

When these preferences conflict, General Motors management and employees should seek a reasonable resolution consistent with GM's respect for the individual.

Each General Motors unit should form a representative task force to implement this policy. The following general guidelines should be taken into consideration:

- In offices, work areas and other facilities where space is shared by two or more employees, an effort shall be made to accommodate individual preferences to the degree practicable.
- In conference rooms and classrooms, etc. smoking is discouraged. Breaks and appropriate access to public areas may be scheduled to accommodate the wishes of smokers.

- In cafeterias, dining areas, and employee lounges, smoking shall be permitted only in identified smoking sections.
- What is anticipated in the foregoing is a spirit of consideration and accommodation rather than substantial changes in facilities.

To address the health concerns of employees, education and smoking cessation programs can be arranged by Medical or Personnel Departments.

This policy does not supersede provision of collective bargaining agreements or posted shop rules and established guidelines for employee conduct concerning controlled or illicit substances, nor does it alter non-smoking areas designated by law.

THE GREYHOUND CORPORATION

The Greyhound Corporation, headquarterd in Phoenix, Arizona, is a diversified company with operations in four principal business segments: *consumer products*, *services*, *transportation manufacturing*, and *financial*. Consumer products are manufactured and marketed by The Dial Corporation, a company that produces leading brands of bar soaps such as Dial and Tone; foods, which include Armour Star Vienna Sausage, Chili and Lunch Bucket microwavable meals; and laundry/household products like Brillo and Purex laundry products. The services facet is comprised of companies such as Dobbs International Services, preparer of inflight meals; Greyhound Airport Services Companies; Travelers Express, the country's leading processor of share drafts; and Greyhound Leisure Services, which operates the Official Cruise Line of Walt Disney World, Premier Cruise Lines. The transportation manufacturing segment builds intercity and transit buses. The financial segment, Greyhound Financial Corporation and Greyhound European Financial Group, provides asset-based financing to mid-sized companies.

Reprinted courtesy of Greyhound Corporation and Angela Phoenix.

Greyhound was formed in 1914 in Hibbing, Minnesota, to transport miners to the Mesabi Iron Range, with the current name being adopted in 1930. In 1971 Greyhound's corporate headquarters were moved to Phoenix, Arizona, a location famous for its low humidity and mild, warm winters. As the result of a diversifying process begun in the '60s to reduce its dependence on intercity bus services, its nationwide transportation company, Greyhound Lines, was sold in 1987. Today, Greyhound Corporation is focused on growth in the consumer products and services businesses and improved profitability in its transportation manufacturing and financial businesses. Construction on the company's new world headquarters, Greyhound Corporate Center, began in May 1989. Greyhound employees will enjoy a pleasant working environment with virtually every feature necessary for efficient business operations. Situated on a prime six acres in the heart of The Phoenix Arts District, the 24-floor twin towers and surrounding environment promise to set a new standard in office space with a masterful marriage of elegance and surroundings conducive to productivity. Among many other special amenities, the new headquarters will feature a 200-seat performing arts center; a health and fitness center and outside a two-acre mini Central Park, providing a tranquil, relaxing retreat. Greyhound Corporation's 1988 revenues were $3.3 billion. Employees in the headquarters and nationwide total approximately 33,000.

Outdoor activities are exploited to their fullest in this multi-climate region, and many of the inhabitants of the "Valley of the Sun" enjoy being outdoors year-round. Most of the activities included in The Greyhound Corporation's Wellness Program involve sports which enable participating employees to enjoy more of the great outdoors.

The Greyhound Corporation Wellness Program is a unique plan which includes contests, lectures, free testing and "corporate challenges"—all designed to make employees more health-conscious as well as instill the corporation's belief that a healthy employee is more productive. Under the strong leadership of Chairman John W. Teets, a former body builder, Greyhound has participated in a series of programs which focus on weight reduction, exercise and preventative maintenance. The Corporation's Wellness Program publication, "CHOICES, " was so named to signify the variety of activities it offers employees who know the importance of a healthy body in renewing energy, reducing stress and keeping their weight down. Employees can make choices from among a series of activities which include: aerobics, basketball, bicycling, cross-country skiing, remaining smoke-free for one year, hiking, lectures, racquetball, running/jogging, soccer, swimming, using seat belts and walking. The company encourages team spirit by having employees join together in many of these activities. Aerobics classes held every day after work for employees are so popular that plans are now under way to expand its current space to accommodate the growing numbers of participants.

Stair-climbing is also an encouraged activity within the program. Each of the 20 floors of Greyhound Tower is marked with signs indicating the number of stairs from floor to lobby. Employees utilizing the stairs in the morning are likely to encounter Chairman Teets making a daily climb to his 19th-floor office.

Special events such as 10K runs are a vital part of the Corporate Wellness Program. For the past nine years, Greyhound has sponsored a 10K run to benefit local charities such as The Muscular Dystrophy Association, The Cystic Fibrosis Center and The Valley of the Sun Hospice, an organization which helps the terminally ill. More than 100 company teams and 3,000 runners participate. Greyhound's race is unique because all entry fees are donated to charity. Almost $150,000 has been raised in recent years.

To encourage a healthy work environment, Greyhound, in 1986, was one of the first major corporations to prohibit smoking within the headquarters building. Free Smoking Cessation Classes and other self-help programs were held in conjunction with a local hospital's health service branch to assist employees and their spouses in "kicking the habit."

A Wellness Check Center was installed in the employee cafeteria with equipment to check blood pressure and heart rate. A computerized scale analyzes ideal weight based on height, sex, age, and build, providing information on the suggested caloric intake to achieve one's desired weight. Literature announcing free immunizations and other health maintenance programs is also available, as well as resource material addressing hypertension, smoking and proper nutrition.

Substance abuse, ranging from alcohol to prescription and illegal drugs, costs organizations billions of dollars a year in med-

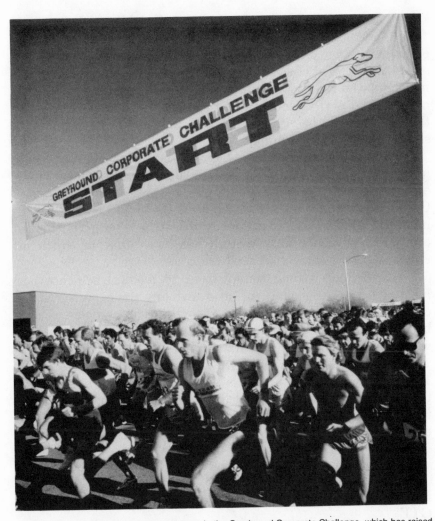

Thousands of runners participate each year in the Greyhound Corporate Challenge, which has raised over $136,000 for charity.

ical expenses and lost productivity. Greyhound believes that education is the key to eliminating such losses and has established Substance Abuse Awareness Sessions to assist employees in their battle against drugs. Another program, Greyhound's Employee Assistance Program, provides trained, certified therapists to counsel employees on stress, work, family, money or drug/alcohol-related problems. Complete confidentiality is a major strength of this program.

Another special feature of Greyhound's Wellness Program is "The Greyhound 600 Club, " a campaign designed to encourage employees to complete a minimum of 100 minutes of weekly exercise for a period of six consecutive weeks. Awards are given to members who reach 600 points. Employees may choose any three activities to earn points. Health-conscious employees attaining these goals have been awarded cash, weekend trips, cruises, T-shirts and exercise equipment.

Weight Watchers, M.I.N.D. Over Weight and other self-help programs provide employees with the opportunity to lose weight at half the cost of outside programs. Through its rebate system, Greyhound employees are eligible for up to $50 or 50% in rebates on all fitness programs. A rebate is also given for an annual physical exam or overall health evaluation which includes tests for cholesterol and triglycerides.

Greyhound's strong commitment to medical self-care and lifestyle management has included utilizing the expertise of top consultants like Dr. Art Mollen. Over the years, employees have benefitted from the wealth of knowledge provided by these experts who specialize in health maintenance and preventive care. In 1987, this commitment won Greyhound the grand prize of the 1987 "Taking Care of Business Award, " presented annually by the Center for Corporate Health Promotion. Greyhound believes that healthy employees can better meet the challenges of the future . . . but it's up to them to make the right *choices*.

GTE

GTE is a worldwide corporation with combined revenues and sales totaling $15.4 billion in 1987. Its three core businesses—telecommunications, lighting and precision materials—employ approximately 161,000 people in 48 states and 33 countries.

Reprinted courtesy of GTE.

In order for GTE to exceed in these core business areas, it cannot be done without GTE's greatest strengths—its employees. GTE's future success depends upon their continued pride and commitment.

To gain this continued commitment, GTE recognizes the importance of establishing a healthy work environment. GTE believes that a healthy employee is a more productive and committed employee. GTE, corporate-wide, is committed to enhancing the health of its employees by providing services such as fitness and wellness programs for its employees.

This is exemplified by the recent development of fitness and wellness programs over a five-year period in seven different locations throughout the country.

Even though each location acts autonomously and decisions are made at the local level, the overall goal is to improve employee well-being.

GTE Corporate Headquarters, located in Stamford, CT, is proud of its fitness and wellness program. We feel that the following description of our program describes the framework that is shared by our other sites corporate-wide.

GTE's philosophy is simply stated, "GTE . . . Working Together to be the Best." The last four words, "to be the Best" represent GTE's objectives to be as good as or better than the best competitor in each market it serves. The first three words, "GTE . . . Working Together," represent the way this objective is achieved.

In upholding this philosophy, the wellness program, under the Department of Health Services, is a prime force. The department is comprised of the Fitness Program, Medical Department and Employee Assistance Program, all working together to enable GTE employees to function at optimal level to be the best.

This could not be accomplished without the establishment of the Wellness Team. Team members of the department include: the Vice-President and Corporate Medical Director, the Health Promotion Coordinator, the Manager of Health and Fitness Programs, four Exercise Specialists, the Corporate Nurse Supervisor, the Occupational Nurse, and the Employee Assistance Manager.

With the comprehensiveness of the Fitness and Wellness Program, the employee is provided with resources to choose from to further improve life-style and to potentially reduce the risk of disease.

Since GTE's inception of its fitness program in February of 1983, the employee has available to him or her the "state-of-the-art" fitness center known to our employees as the MET (Medical Exercise Training Facility). The cost to the employee is only a few dollars per paycheck.

The MET is comprised of a 9,237-square-foot facility including an aerobics room, main exercise floor, fitness evaluation laboratory, and men's and women's locker rooms.

The aerobics room is approximately 900 square feet and is used for various types of exercise classes for employees interested in group exercise programs.

For the employee interested in individual exercise, he or she can participate in the MET exercise program. The exercise facility is 3,500 square feet and is equipped with 6 Monarch stationary bicycle ergometers, 10 individual pieces of Keiser muscle strengthening machines, 3 Concept II rowing ergometers, 1 Cybex upper body ergometer, 2 PT 4000 Stairmasters and 7 Quinton treadmills.

Before employees can enter the fitness program, they must complete a medical history and health evaluation.

Following this procedure, a comprehensive and confidential health risk appraisal is taken which will estimate the risk of disease over a ten-year period (coronary heart disease, cerebral vascular disease, cancer and risk of injury).

Once the employee completes the health risk appraisal, he or she is then brought through a fitness evaluation that measures the parameters of blood pressure, flexibility, body composition and cardiovascular assessment. The results of this information serve as a basis for the exercise prescription that is designed by the exercise specialist.

The success of our Fitness and Wellness programs is attributed to the quality of our fitness staff whose responsibilities are to teach our ongoing health education programs. The fitness staff is exceptional in their talent and expertise, all holding an advanced degree in the health and fitness field.

For the past five years, GTE's commitment to its employees' health goes beyond the doors of the fitness center. Realizing that fitness is one part of the wellness picture, the development of the Health Education program called "Bright Life" is of equal importance.

Our health, which many of us take for granted, is our most important possession. Good health depends on a number of factors, including heredity, life-style (i.e., diet and exercise), environment and personality traits (i.e., attitude toward life, self and work). Because 50% or more of illness and early death is attributed to life-style, GTE recognizes the value of educating its employees on the potential hazards of associate risk factors—smoking, lack of exercise, poor nutrition, obesity, alcohol intake, and not using the seat belt.

These risk factors can be identified through the health risk appraisal and the employee has the opportunity to improve his health and well-being by choosing from our Bright Life Program. The Bright Life Programs include the following courses:

1. Nutrition (called the SENSE program).
2. Weight control (called "Pounds Off").
3. Healthy Back Program.
4. Stress Management (called "Coping with Change").
5. Smoking Cessation.
6. Cardio-pulmonary Resuscitation.
7. First-aid.
8. Health Risk Appraisal.
9. Breast Self-Examination.

The intent of these courses under the "Bright Life" philosophy is to help employees become aware of their own habits that later may affect their health. It is the goal of GTE's wellness program that each employee who participates will gain the confidence and education and skills to identify negative health habits to enhance his or her life-style.

HALLMARK CARDS, INC.

Hallmark Cards, Inc., the world's largest greeting card company, traces its beginning to January 10, 1910 when Joyce C. Hall, then an 18-year-old from Norfolk, Nebraska, arrived at the train station in Kansas City. Armed only with an inventory consisting of two shoe boxes full of picture postcards, he quickly began selling to retailers throughout the Midwest. Success followed and soon the teenage businessman had cleared $200 and opened a checking account. In 1912, a year after brother Rollie joined him, Joyce Hall added greeting cards to the line, and by 1915 the brothers had begun making some of their own cards.

In 1954, the Hall Brothers firm officially changed its name to Hallmark, and today more than 80 years since its beginnings, Hallmark employs 20,000 full-time employees world-wide. In addition to greeting cards (more than 11 million are produced each day), Hallmark manufactures calendars, gift wrap, party goods, plush toys, jigsaw puzzles, home decorations and a host of other social expression products. Products are published in more than 20 languages and distributed in more than 100 countries under the brand names of Hallmark, Ambassador, Springbok, Crayola, Liquitex, and Heartline. With annual sales in excess of $2.3 billion, this privately held company would rank near the middle of the Fortune 500 list of publicly held industrial concerns.

From its earliest days, Hallmark has been concerned with quality—a quality that extends beyond its products and services to its sponsorship of the Emmy-award-winning Hallmark Hall of Fame (the longest-running dramatic playhouse in the history of television) and to its slogan, "When you care enough to send the very best, " one of the most believed slogans in America.

This commitment to excellence also has been evident in Hallmark's employee benefit programs. When, in 1956, the company introduced the Hallmark Career Rewards Program to its employees, *Fortune* magazine called it "the country's most liberal employee-benefit and profit-sharing plan." And in 1984 and again in 1987, Hallmark was selected as one of the country's top 10

Reprinted courtesy of Hallmark Cards, Inc.

employers in the book, *The 100 Best Companies to Work for in America.* For the last two years, *Working Mother* magazine has selected Hallmark as one of "The Best Companies for Working Mothers."

This concern for the health and well-being of its employees is the philosophy that prompted Hallmark to develop "Healthworks, " a wellness program that combines company capabilities with community resources. The goal of Healthworks is to increase employees' awareness that healthy lifestyles bring happier, more productive, and possibly longer, lives.

By focusing on several components of wellness—health, fitness, safety and environment, recreation, nutrition and employee assistance—Healthworks provides a comprehensive approach to wellness.

Health:　Providing for employees' health care needs is an integral part of Healthworks. The Hallmark Medical Department offers a variety of services, including emergency care for those injured or who became ill at work, physical therapy, allergy injections and evaluation of medical conditions. In addition, emphasis is placed on the prevention of disease and accidents through health education programs. Classes are offered in first aid, CPR, weight loss, smoking cessation, nutrition, stress management and back injury prevention. Blood pressure testing and hearing/vision screening also are available. At the Kansas City headquarters, smoking is not permitted except in designated areas; cigarette vending machines were removed recently as a means of further promoting good health.

Fitness:　The Hallmark fitness center, located adjacent to the corporate headquarters building, opened in 1980. The 14,000-square-foot facility features a banked 1/18-mile running track, an aerobics room and gym, a variety of state-of-the-art electronic exercise equipment, and shower and locker facilities. Modern, synthetic sport surfaces have been installed throughout the fitness center to lessen the possibility of injury and to enhance fitness programs. Numerous aerobic and other organized fitness programs are offered five days a week, before and after work hours. More than 2,000 corporate employees have signed up to use the center.

Recreation: Recreational sports at Hallmark began in 1924 when the first women's basketball team was organized. Today, more than 2,220 employees participate in company-sponsored softball, basketball, volleyball, soccer, tennis, bowling and golf leagues. The most popular activity is softball, with more than 50 teams and 700 employees participating each summer. In addition, Hallmark employees compete in the annual Kansas City Corporate challenge, a major sporting event that involves companies from throughout the Kansas City area. The availability of these recreational activities not only inspires employees to stay in good physical condition year-round, but also boosts morale and enhances working relationships.

Nutrition: Hallmark has emphasized healthy, nutritional foods since the company's cafeteria service began in 1924. To encourage employees to develop and maintain healthy eating habits, the headquarters cafeteria provides a daily selection of "light" menu items as well as typed menus that feature the number of calories contained with each food item. In addition, food measured by the ounce in the cafeteria deli offers frozen and fresh yogurt along with fresh fruit. Special events, such as Valentine's Day's "Be Good to your Heart" lunch program, promote positive eating practices by offering low-sodium, low-cholesterol and low-fat menu choices.

Safety & Environment: To maintain safety on the job, Hallmark monitors and analyzes the work environment on a regular basis. Studies are conducted at all Hallmark facilities to determine safe levels of noise, temperature, and lighting. In addition, Hallmark's Advanced Technical Research laboratory can sample atmospheres and report exposures to chemicals for both short-term and eight-hour work periods. Sensitive scales can weigh minute amounts of particles that are gathered from air samplings.

Employee Assistance: Providing confidential assistance is a vital part of Hallmark's concern for its employees. With the objective of improving the quality of life off the job as well as on the job, confidential employee counseling is available to help identify a variety of resources related to the employee's specific needs. Employees can obtain advice and referral in regard to family conflicts, alcohol or drug problems, career opportunities and financial concerns. Since 1986, a program called "Family Care Choices" has been available to help employees locate care providers for their children, aging parents and disabled family members. In 1988, Hallmark introduced a professional counseling service that offers the assistance of three Kansas City psychologists to employees in times of personal crisis.

All of these components working together have made Healthworks an unqualified success. The program has and continues to enjoy excellent response and participation among employees. With Healthworks, Hallmark continues its commitment to excellence by providing employees the opportunity to achieve a better quality life.

HEWLETT-PACKARD COMPANY

Hewlett-Packard Company, headquartered in Palo Alto, California, makes computing and electronic measuring equipment for people in business, industry, science, engineering, health care and education. HP's more than 10,000 products include integrated instrument and computer systems, test and measuring instruments, computer systems and peripheral products, handheld calculators, medical electronic equipment and instrumentation and systems for chemical analysis.

HP is one of the 100 largest industrial corporations in America, with revenue of $9.8 billion and earnings of $816 million in its 1988 fiscal year (ended October 31). The company employs 87,000 people, of whom 56,000 work in the U.S. HP plants are located in 24 U.S. cities, most of which are in California, Colorado, the Northeast and Pacific Northwest. The company also has research and manufacturing facilities in Europe, Japan, Latin America and Canada, and manufacturing operations in Southeast Asia.

Reprinted courtesy of Hewlett-Packard Company.

Since Hewlett-Packard is organized into more than 50 entities which maintain a degree of autonomy, wellness programs vary. Companywide, HP offers flexible working hours, allowing most employees to start their work day between 6:00 and 9:00 in the morning and finish eight hours later. This policy provides greater freedom in scheduling personal activities, such as an exercise program, at times that are most convenient for employees.

Many HP sites feature one or more exercise areas, such as basketball courts, softball diamonds and running courses. These sites also offer locker rooms and showers for use by employees. Individual entities sponsor in-house classes in aerobics, stress management, nutrition and other wellness topics. Some entities have exercise equipment on site for employees' use.

A confidential Employee Assistance Program (EAP) is available to Hewlett-Packard employees and their eligible dependents who may be suffering from personal or family problems.

Several entities have developed their own aggressive programs to promote employee wellness. HP's site in Boise, Idaho, has taught a wellness course to more than one-third of their employee population during the past year. The class, called "Take Charge," is co-led by a nurse, and includes segments on getting more information from your doctor and better maintaining your own health. Many HP entities sponsor annual health fairs at which community organizations, such as hospitals and health associations, staff booths to educate employees about wellness issues.

Registered nurses maintain an office at all HP sites.

HOLIDAY CORPORATION

In 1982, Holiday Corporation opened its 17,000-square-foot fitness center on the grounds of its Holiday Inns, Inc. headquarters offices in Memphis, Tenn. The facility has since become the centerpiece of a multi-faceted health and wellness program for the company's employees.

Reprinted courtesy of Holiday Corporation.

The overall mission of the fitness and health promotion effort of the Corporation is: To provide Holiday Corporation employees and their families with the opportunity, incentives, and support to live and work in a healthy and productive manner. Based on a comprehensive approach to wellness, a solid foundation for achieving this mission with our headquarters employees is in place.

From the beginning health promotion and the related fitness and wellness efforts have been characterized by strong leadership, support, and involvement by senior management, and a high level of involvement by employees from all departments and locations.

The fitness center itself is one of the most complete facilities in the city of Memphis (see facility description). Employees may use the center during any regularly scheduled hours, and family members may use the facility, equipment and classes on a slightly restricted schedule. There is no fee. One guest is allowed to accompany an employee. However, in the years since its opening, programs have expanded beyond the walls of the center and are now reaching those employees not inclined to use such a benefit.

The first step beyond the walls of the facility was into recreational sports such as volleyball, walleyball, racquetball, golf tournaments, a running team and tennis leagues. A strong recreational component has been helpful in attracting a variety of people who like to combine activity with competition and with social interaction. Recreation programs also provide an excellent method for people from various departments and levels within the company to meet and mix in a non-traditional business forum. The recreational programs are now firmly entrenched in the headquarters' culture with approximately 25 percent of the headquarters employees participating in at least one activity each year.

The next step beyond the typical fitness programs was into the area of food and diet. A low-fat entree program called "Rick's-Picks," selected by the director of the fitness center, selects one meal low-in-fat in the employee cafeteria each afternoon. The program has been so well received by employees that the low-fat entree is the cafeteria's best selling lunch item daily.

The concept of diet and weight control hit national levels in 1988 when the fitness center staff sponsored the Holiday Corporation National Mid-Winter Meltdown. The weight loss program challenged teams of ten employees each to lose up to 20 pounds per employee over a 60-day period. A weight control pamphlet and diet guide, T-shirts and refrigerator magnets helped lead the company to a total weight loss of over 10 tons. Approximately 10 percent of the company's employees participated in the effort. The program was repeated in 1989 with similar success.

General wellness and health awareness programs have become a center of attention at the Holiday Corporation fitness center over the last few years. A clean-air policy was implemented in 1987 at all headquarters buildings. The policy phased in a smoke-free office environment. Health screening programs are offered on a regular basis for headquarters employees. The programs address such issues as blood pressure, cholesterol, mammography and general health awareness. Wellness and health education are also incorporated into company training programs and offered as stand-alone classes throughout the year. Finally, all of the programs and issues are communicated to employees through a monthly fitness center newsletter.

At the fitness center, employees are given an opportunity to address their personal health and fitness needs or goals through a personalized exercise prescription. It begins with a required "fit check" when a new employee or family member joins the center. This "fit check," conducted in the center's fitness testing lab, looks at medical history, interests, resting heart rate and blood pressure, body fat analysis for projection of target weight, aerobic fitness testing, and strength and flexibility testing. The information gathered is used to develop an individual's personalized exercise prescription for health improvement and for measuring health and fitness progress. The assessments are also available upon request.

As the fitness and wellness programs at Holiday Corporation look to the future, the role is expanding to achieve the results seen at the headquarters offices to the approximately 40,000 employees working in Holiday Inn, Hampton Inn, Embassy Suites, Homewood Suites and Harrah's hotel and casino/hotel locations across the country. The National Mid-Winter Meltdown was the first effort in this plan.

Not only does Holiday Corporation expect to expand its fitness programs to all of its employees, but plans are also underway to link health promotion to health insurance and cost containment efforts. By treating health promotion as a human resources management tool, we believe we can create a supportive environment for healthy lifestyle choices, while helping our employees develop skills for healthy living.

STAFF

Manager, Health Promotion: Responsible for the overall operation of the fitness center, developing national programs and linking health promotion with health cost containment.

Supervisor, Fitness and Health Services: Responsible for the day-to-day activities of the fitness center and related programs.

Health Services Administrator: Responsible for the employee health clinic and is involved with special programs, seminars and health screenings. The administrator is the editor of the monthly newsletter and is responsible for the highly successful aerobics programs.

Fitness Center Coordinator: Responsible for running the fitness center office. Also responsible for scheduling company executive physicals, producing the newsletter, coordinating special projects, new employee orientation, registration, membership data and scheduling of court time.

Health/Fitness Specialist: Responsible for fitness testing, exercise prescription, exercise instruction and special projects.

In addition, a part-time staff of aerobic instructors teach 15 classes each week. Four faculty monitors assist during peak hours and interns are hired on a regular basis.

Facilities (17,000-square-foot total area)

three racquetball courts
1,900-square-foot aerobics area with suspended wooden floor
1,200-square-foot exercise area, including:
    seven treadmills
    10 stationary bikes

two rowing machines
two stair climbing machines
a free weight area
gravitron
a Keiser Strength Training Circuit
sauna/whirlpool
indoor swimming pool
four lighted tennis courts
a half-mile rubberized, lighted walk/jog trail
volleyball courts
picnic area

HOME BOX OFFICE

The reasons for participating in the Fitness Center program are many. Medically, there are direct, positive benefits in terms of cardiovascular physiology. The right type and intensity of exercise will assist in controlling components of the blood that relate to atherosclerosis and diabetes mellitus. In addition, exercise is extremely effective in assisting in weight control and can be beneficial in eliminating the negative stresses we all confront in our daily lives.

FITNESS CENTER LOCATION/DESCRIPTION

The Fitness Center is on Grace 2 in the Southwest corner, with a splendid view of Bryant Park. It is approximately 2,900 square feet in size and is divided into a reception area, men's and women's dressing rooms, squash court, circuit training area and an office for staff use. The circuit training area is stocked with treadmills, Stairmasters, a UBE, bicycles, free weights, cross country skis, and a full line of muscular conditioning equipment from Eagle. Additionally, there are instructor-led aerobic, yoga, and back

Reprinted courtesy of Home Box Office.

care classes, as well as squash and basketball play throughout the week. Once you are oriented to the program, you will be assigned a locker for storage of your exercise shoes. Freshly laundered uniforms, towels and toiletries will be provided daily.

PROGRAM DESCRIPTION

The Fitness Program will be individually tailored to the needs and desires of each participant. Prior to entrance, a comprehensive screening process will be conducted that will appraise each participant's coronary risk through a blood chemistry analysis and a health history questionnaire. Based on the results of these tests, participants will then undergo a cardiovascular functional evaluation. A battery of physical fitness assessments will then be the final phase of entry screening for all participants.

There are two initial purposes for these tests—first, to determine if there are any cardiovascular concerns that may preclude exercise; and second, to determine aerobic or endurance capabilities.

Once the screening procedures have been successfully completed, the daily exercise routine will vary depending on each participant's capabilities and preferences. The workout options are as follows:

Circuit Training. Utilizing the equipment mentioned previously, a circuit workout will be set up for all participants as the mainstay of the program. In a circuit workout, one moves quickly from one piece of equipment to another, working on both endurance and muscular conditioning. At each station the workload should be adjusted to the capabilities of the individual.

Class Activities. Classes offered and time schedules will depend, to a large extent, on participant needs. Class options presently include the following:

High Energy Aerobics
Low Impact Aerobics
Total Toning

Stretch and Flex
Self Defense
HBO Back School

Squash. During certain hours the squash court will be available for scheduled play. Reservations should be made in advance. A squash instructor is available for individual lessons. Call Roger Wooden at X8163 to reserve court time. We supply all equipment for regular play.

Basketball. There is regularly scheduled basketball Monday through Friday. Play is restricted to a maximum number of six players at a time on a first come, first served basis.

Hours. The Fitness Center will be open for use Monday through Friday, 7 A.M. until 9:30 A.M. and closing 9:30 A.M. until 11:30 A.M. Afternoon hours run straight through from 11:30 A.M. until 7:30 P.M. From 7:30 P.M. until 9:00 P.M. the Center will remain open to those members on the late-night list; however, it will be unsupervised by staff members.
Participants who wish to work out during the unattended hours need clearance from the staff. This will be solely for the purpose of insuring your safety and proper use of the equipment. The guard at the front door will not admit anyone who has not been previously cleared. If you are interested in working out during these hours, please contact a staff member for clearance.

Staff. The staff consists of two exercise specialists, Bill Boyle and Gail Trojack. Roger Wooden is facility attendant. Bill and Gail have advanced degrees in exercise science and adult fitness management. They bring to the program experience in group exercise, aerobic and weight training and testing, as well as expertise in health education and counseling.
There will be a fee to use the Fitness Center, collected through a payroll deduction of $7 per pay period. Deductions will begin one month after you start exercising. Your first month is free!

IBM

IBM has instituted prevention-oriented health programs for employees and their families to help improve participants' health and curb spiraling health-care costs. The Wellness programs provide a wide range of company-sponsored courses and activities, most of which are free of charge to participants.

Because of the number of employees, the Wellness program is decentralized to a large extent. Implementation and communication are the responsibility of local managers, but basically the same programs are offered for all employees at all locations. In order to design and administer the programs as effectively as possible, the company frequently uses outside specialists to provide a high level of services and continuous improvements.

A PLAN FOR LIFE

In 1981, IBM launched A Plan for Life (APFL), a health education program designed to give employees and their families information on and support for healthier lifestyles. The objective of the program is to encourage employees and their families to take personal responsibility for their health.

APFL offers a comprehensive array of courses on popular subjects such as exercise, weight management, cardiopulmonary resuscitation (CPR), and defensive driving. Most courses last from two to twelve weeks and are taught by qualified instructors affiliated with organizations such as YMCA, YWCA, American Cancer Society, American Red Cross, hospitals and colleges.

APFL is typical of the company's approach to wellness by providing quality offerings at locations across the country on a voluntary basis. All IBM regular and retired employees and their spouses and dependent children aged 15–22 are eligible to partic-

Reprinted courtesy of IBM.

ipate in company-paid and sponsored courses. In addition, individuals may enroll in similar qualified courses provided by community or commercial organizations on a tuition assistance basis.

VOLUNTARY HEALTH ASSESSMENT

The gradual shift of IBM programs toward an emphasis on wellness or preventive health care is illustrated clearly by the Voluntary Health Assessment (VHA), which was introduced by the company in 1986 as a successor to its Voluntary Health Screening Program in effect since 1985. VHA is offered at five-year intervals to all IBM employees age 25 or over, and the company expects to give about 35,000 examinations per year under the program.

Instead of merely identifying disease, the VHA generates a health profile for each employee based on age, lifestyle, heredity and other pertinent personal information. It then identifies an individual's risk of developing a particular illness and suggests steps the person can take to significantly lower that risk.

EMPLOYEE ASSISTANCE PROGRAM

The IBM Employee Assistance Program (EAP) was introduced in 1984 to provide prompt, professional and private counseling for emotional concerns, marital and family difficulties, and problems relating to alcohol or other drug use. An IBM employee, retiree or eligible dependent may receive, at no cost, up to eight visits with an EAP counselor for problem assessment and short-term counseling. For specialized or longer-term problems, referrals may be made to prescreened community resources.

EAP service is offered through two leading firms that specialize in providing service to corporate clients. The design of IBM's EAP includes an unusually comprehensive evaluation process that monitors usage, client satisfaction and quality while maintaining the client confidentiality that is central to the program.

IBM's EAP fits within the wellness or prevention framework espoused by the company because it offers an immediate source of professional help and referral before everyday programs become overwhelming.

An innovative aspect of IBM's EAP is the availability of a voluntary network of IBM employees and retirees to provide support and encouragement to other employees and retirees suffering from alcoholism. The network includes individuals who have had experience in coping with the alcohol-related problems of others as well as those who have had problems themselves.

MEDICAL BENEFITS/PERSONAL HEALTH ACCOUNT

Along with its preventive programs, IBM offers a comprehensive medical benefits plan to address the health care and treatment needs of its employees and their families. The plan includes coverage for major medical expenses, surgery, hospitalization and dental care.

In 1985, a benefit called the Personal Health Account (PHA) was added to IBM's medical plan. It provides financial assistance for preventive care that can keep people healthier and lower long-term medical costs. Examples of PHA coverage are procedures such as Pap smears and mammograms for women, preventive tests for blood sugar and cholesterol level, well baby care, hearing care, eye examinations and corrective lenses, and various immunizations.

OFF-THE-JOB SAFETY

Because most serious injuries occur off the job, IBM provides extensive and frequent information to employees and their families on home safety, safe driving and health-related safety.

All of IBM's wellness programs are designed to interrelate with one another. For example, as individuals are made aware of health risks through the Voluntary Health Assessment or A Plan for Life, they can then use the Personal Health Account to help pay for preventive measures that can help safeguard against those risks and avoid future problems. Or, the Employee Assistance Program may result in enrollment in a course in stress management offered through A Plan for Life. And, reports from the Voluntary Health Assessment cover risk of injury in an automobile accident—risk that can be lowered by wearing a seat belt.

IBM's wellness programs emphasize a healthier lifestyle that can help prevent sickness before it begins and increase the capacity to recover more quickly if illness does strike. The company's wellness programs reflect its belief that healthy employees are more productive, use fewer medical benefits, and thus slow the escalating costs of health care.

ICI AMERICAS INC.

ICI Americas Inc., the U.S. operating subsidiary for Imperial Chemical Industries PLC, of London, England, is headquartered in Wilmington, Delaware. The Company employs over 18,000 men and women in the U.S. and has sales in excess of $3 billion.

ICI is comprised of nine business groups: ICI Advanced Materials, ICI Agricultural Products, ICI Electronics, ICI Films, ICI General Products, ICI Glidden, ICI Pharmaceuticals, ICI Polyurethanes and ICI Specialty Chemicals. These Groups are supported by corporate staff services including Employee Relations and Administration, Finance, Law, Secretary's, Public Affairs, Purchasing and Distribution and Technology and Strategy.

The Company has research and development laboratories, sales offices and over 50 manufacturing facilities strategically located throughout the U.S.

The ICI Americas Center for Health and Fitness offers a comprehensive program for all employees at its headquarters complex: individual and group exercise programs, health risk appraisals

Reprinted courtesy of ICI Americas, Inc.

and lifestyle enhancement programs such as smoking cessation, stress management, nutrition and CPR training. The facility and programs are designed to encourage lifestyle strategies that lead to personal well-being.

The Center is managed by qualified fitness professionals with education, training and experience in physical fitness and exercise physiology. The staff is working under the direction of a physician in the Corporate Medical Group.

The 5,000 square feet facility is divided into five areas.

The cardiovascular exercise room is equipped with five Bodyguard bicycles, two Biocycles, four Schwinn Airdynes, four Marquette treadmills, two Concept II rowers, and one Nordic track skier. A ten station circuit of Keiser strength equipment, two Universal kick pulleys, and a set of Universal dumbbells outfit the muscular strength and endurance room.

The remaining areas include two locker rooms and a multipurpose room used for exercise classes, wellness programs, lifestyle modification courses, and fitness assessments.

All employees at the ICI headquarters complex are eligible to use the Center. In order to participate in the program all must go through medical screening and fitness testing, depending upon variables such as age, medical risk factors, and health status. The screening program is designed to promote the safe use of the facility and its programs. Each member is given an individualized computer-generated exercise program based on health history, fitness objectives and the results of baseline physiological tests. Follow-up testing at six-month intervals documents progress and provides additional opportunities for motivation and education.

Each registered participant receives a pair of shorts, T-shirt (with logo), clean towels, soap and shampoo. Hair dryers are available in the grooming areas of the locker rooms.

Membership in early 1989 numbers over 700. There are approximately 2,500 employees at the headquarters complex. The current cost of participation to the employees in the program is $9.00 per month. The Center is open from 6:00 A.M.–7:00 P.M. Monday–Friday, and 8:00 A.M.–12 noon on Saturday. Those employees who have identified medical risk factors, with the permission of their immediate supervisors, may use the facility during mid-day or morning hours. All other employees are encouraged to arrange their personal schedules to use the Center either at lunch, before or after normal work hours.

Modified wellness programs have been established at other ICIA sites. They range from an exercise room to lifestyle modification courses such as smoking cessation, aerobics, weight reduction, jogging, and good nutrition.

JOSTENS

Since its founding in 1897 as a small watch repair shop in Owatonna, Minnesota, Jostens has grown to a large diversified company with facilities across the United States and Canada. Today, as a leading provider of products and services for the youth, education, sports award and recognition markets, Jostens has seven operating divisions and annual sales of more than $500 million and has been on the "Fortune 500" list of largest publicly held U.S. industrial corporations since 1985. Jostens supplied the medals for the 1984 Summer Olympics and its Canadian subsidiary manufactured the medals for the 1988 Olympics Winter Games.

The company, with approximately 7,000 employees and 1,200 independent sales representatives and 34 plant and office facilities, is headquartered in Minneapolis, Minnesota. The seven operating divisions, their locations and products are as follows:

Scholastic—Porterville, CA; Santa Barbara, CA; Attleboro, MA; Owatonna, MN; Red Wing, MN; Laurens, SC; Shelbyville, TN and Denton, TX.—High School and college class rings, graduation announcements and diplomas, trophies and awards, graduation caps and gowns.

Printing and Publishing—Visalia, CA; Topeka, KS; State College, PA and Clarksville, TN and Hunter Publishing, Winston Salem, NC.—High School and college yearbooks, commercial publications.

Reprinted courtesy of Jostens.

Artex—Abilene, KS; Boonville, KS; Manhattan, KS; Overland Park, KS and Yates Center, KS.—Custom-imprinted activewear.

Recognition—Princeton, IL; Rochester, MI; Omaha, NE and Memphis, TN.—Custom-designed rings and jewelry; silver, crystal and other gifts; plaques and certificates.

Education—Phoenix, AZ; Springfield, IL and San Diego, CA.—Customized computer-based learning labs, computer software and hardware for classroom instruction, audio-visual learning aids.

Canada—Winnipeg, Manitoba; Missisauga, Ontario; Lachine, Quebec and Sherbrook, Quebec.—Class rings, yearbooks, school photography, recognition awards.

Wayneco—Wayne, PA.—Direct marketing of premium and limited edition products to university alumni and other special groups.

Any company's success story and the mutually satisfying relationship between employee and employer is one to be nurtured to meet the delicate balance of employee needs and the needs of the organization. Achieving this balance is an ongoing challenge which Jostens is meeting by offering its employees opportunities to excel and achieve excellence in most facets of their lives.

Jostens has joined many other corporations in the effort to increase employees' awareness of the role of good health in their lives. The development of a "Wellness Program" was begun in incremental steps designed to heighten awareness to the impact of health on the whole of one's life, to include work, home life, school and other interactions, and activities.

In 1984 the company began subscribing to *Your Health & Fitness*, published by General Learning Corporation. This bimonthly still goes to every Jostens employee and independent sales agent across the country. Chosen from among several outstanding publications to be one of the company's vehicles to carry health and fitness information to the workforce, it is sent directly to the employee or sales agent's home. Sharing with the employee's family has been found to be a key ingredient because the health of the whole family is critical to the health and performance of the employee. All of Jostens' wellness programs, therefore, have been and will continue to be open to family members.

In 1984 the company also introduced the Employee Assistance Program. While good physical health is extremely important, so too is the mental health and well-being of each employee and of his or her family members. Our Assistance program is confidential and provides free initial counseling to employees having problems in any of the following areas: family; marital conflicts; relationships; parenting; separation/divorce; emotional/behavioral; alcohol use; drugs; job stress; vocational; grief and loss; day care; legal; tenant's rights; physical abuse; personal financial management; physical health; sexual harrassment; housing; retirement and any other areas causing concern. Employees have access to a 24-hour *Help Line* answered by counselors trained to provide immediate help with crisis problems or to direct employees in non-crisis situations. Employees have a second option which is *In-Person* counseling. In both instances counselors provide employees with problem evaluation and assessment and identify major issues of concern and develop a plan of action for change. This plan is open to all members of employees' or sales agents' families and is provided for by Jostens. If subsequent care is recommended for which there is a charge, those charges, if medical in nature, will most likely be covered by one of the medical plans offered to employees and agents.

Since the company has 36 locations, Jostens has chosen to have a decentralized Wellness effort with each location having imput into what its employees would like to have. The Corporate Human Resources department gives guidance to the plant locations and serves as a resource for specific programs or for obtaining specific information or materials. Local management, primarily the personnel manager at that location, is responsible for the development and implementation of the program.

Jostens prides itself on its history of community involvement and sponsorship of numerous charitable events. For years the company has sponsored events such as the 5K and 10K Kaiser Roll Races where wheelchair racers and able-bodied runners compete side by side. Proceeds from this event go to the American Lung

Association and to other non-profit organizations toward combating disabling diseases. The company is also involved with the Special Olympics on an annual basis and has recently made and donated the medals for this event. In all such efforts, the Jostens community nationwide is encouraged to participate, if not actively, then as well-wishers, and to lend support and enthusiasm for the efforts of those involved. Hand in hand with such events as the Kaiser Roll and the Special Olympics, Jostens employees and management have shown support for community health endeavors through yearly participation in the March of Dimes Team Walk where employees volunteer to walk and their miles are paid for by other employees, neighbors, relatives, friends. Participation is encouraged as employees are not only doing a good deed but are also doing something healthy. This year, 27 headquarters employees participated and their pledges matched by the Jostens Foundation totaled nearly $5,000.00.

At the headquarters location some of the events sponsored have been received with more enthusiasm and employee support than others. Bearing this in mind, the company recognizes that not every program will be subscribed to by each and every employee. The challenge has been to provide employees with opportunities to have input into the activities they want to participate in and then to offer these if possible. One way to determine this interest was to have a company Health Fair with many activities presented under one roof. These fairs (there have been three of them to date) have been successful events with good employee participation. The Wellness committee, staffed by employees, organized and orchestrated each Health Fair. Our most recent, held in the Spring of 1987, boasted the following exhibits and demonstrations: blood pressure checks; blood work-ups for cholesterol and diabetes; body fat compositions testing; height and weight measurements; lung capacity screening; flexibility and bench press testing; therapeutic massage; cancer risk assessment; vision testing; glaucoma testing; fitness equipment demonstrations; literature on exercise, safety, nutrition, smoking risks, etc. These fairs have served as models for our plant locations. Interest surveys issued after each fair have helped the company gear its programs to meet the needs and wants of the workforce. The cost factor associated with presentation of the health fairs was held to a minimum because the Wellness Committee was able to solicit vendor services either gratis or at minimal cost. The committee sought out and received the services of the two HMO's which service our local employees. Eager to assist were also such organizations as the March of Dimes, the American Cancer Society, The American Lung Association, a local Heart Health organization and numerous other organizations who provided personnel, literature and necessary equipment.

The plant locations have followed suit with similar programs designed to fit the local workforce. The plants have followed Jostens' philosophy of service to the community and the workforce has eagerly participated in walkathons, decathalons and other similar activities to help raise needed funding while having fun doing something healthy.

At the headquarters location, the company has provided space for the weekly Josfit meetings which interested employees have arranged on an ongoing basis. This after-hours event is an aerobics/jazzercise class. Employees have contracted with a YMCA instructor to lead the session. The employees pay the instructor, Jostens provides the facility.

The Jostens headquarters avails itself of special rates with two local health club organizations, the Northwest Racquet and Swim Club and the YMCA. Employees may receive special discounted "corporate" rates if they join during specific times and show proof of working at Jostens. In many cases the savings are substantial, up to $400/year. Plants have sought out similar discounted group rates. The company also sponsors employees' sports such as softball, volleyball, basketball, golf, and bowling. Most facilities have provided space for aerobics and stretch classes for all shifts where there is more than one shift.

In virtually every instance where Jostens has promoted better health for its employees, the community in general has benefited. It is natural then that in an arena where many face the greatest personal challenge, namely that of achieving and maintaining a healthy weight level, the company sought a novel way to reward its employees for achievement of a very difficult goal. Last year the Wellness Committee came up with the idea of matching the pounds lost with dollars for the local food shelf. The company offered the Weight Watchers program on-site over the lunch hours and lost pounds rapidly translated into smiles on employees' faces as well as on the faces of officials of the Minnesota Food Share. Employees were charged a co-payment for Weight Watchers. Those who completed all sessions and/or lost the desired excess pounds were issued reimbursement checks. The corporate Wellness group will suggest its program of giving to the needy as one type of reward for future consideration at the plant locations.

The corporate headquarters broke ground in a highly controversial area of wellness, namely the war on smoking. The past three years has seen the gradual elimination of smoking at the headquarters location. The need to be in compliance with the rather stringent Clean-Air Act of Minnesota and the conviction that its employees deserve to enjoy a work environment which is smoke free, led to a 3-year series of events which culminated in a general smoking ban on April 1, 1988. Jostens offered on-site smoking cessation programs as well as partial reimbursement for off-site programs. Those employees who choose to participate in the cessation programs have enjoyed a high measure of success and are already reaping the rewards of this step toward better health. The plant locations are in varying stages with smoking vs. non-smoking. Some have designated *no smoking* areas. Some have restricted smoking to one area (lunch room), some have put no restrictions on smoking. Each location should let employee requests and local ordinances determine the course which that facility should take. Employee buy-in is important for the most positive results.

In conclusion, the Jostens Wellness process has evolved over the past several years. While the company has not erected health spas or converted office space to this effort, great progress has been made toward enlightening its employees to the positives of good health. The company does not take the posture that employee participation is mandatory. Instead, it has chosen the route of providing information and opportunity. Good health is a *shared* responsibility and the rewards to both employees and the company are and will continue to be immense.

K-TRON INTERNATIONAL, INC.

K-Tron International, Inc. is the leading manufacturer of digital measurement products, including process control feeders and loss-in-weight security systems. K-Tron equipment is responsible for putting just the right amount of raisins in your raisin bran, ingredients in your granola bars and whitening power in your detergent. In addition to the more familiar applications in the food industry, K-Tron process control equipment is used by Fortune 500 companies in the chemical, pharmaceutical, plastics and cosmetics industries. The company has been designing, manufacturing and marketing feeders and electronic controllers since 1964, and in 1987 extended its business to include the design and manufacture of security systems. The company applied its expertise in weighing technology to develop a new security system for R.J. Reynolds that detects shoplifting from retail merchandising racks and is currently pursuing additional markets for this new product.

K-Tron has two manufacturing facilities: K-Tron Corporation is located in Pitman, New Jersey and K-Tron Soder is in Niederlenz, Switzerland, near Zurich. Marketing offices are maintained in Rungis, France; Gelnhausen, Germany; and Oldham, England. Another wholly-owned subsidiary, K-Tron International Marketing Corporation, is located in New Jersey and is responsible for marketing products in the Far East and for maintaining a spare parts operation in Hong Kong. K-Tron employs 500 employees world-wide.

Fitness has long been characteristic of Swiss culture and daily life. We all have seen and can easily visualize Swiss mountaineers scaling the Alps! Walking is a way of life even today. And fitness is as important as ever. In 1987 K-Tron Soder built a 4-story administration building adjacent to its manufacturing facility. The lower level of this new building is used for meetings, training classes, and has an exclusive fitness center for employees. Exercise classes for employees are currently held

---

Reprinted courtesy of K-Tron International, Inc.

there and future planning includes the addition of exercise equipment. The building was built with men's and women's showers installed there in anticipation of expanding K-Tron Soder's "Fitness Program." The company has also contributed towards the purchase of a chalet to be used by employees and their families for ski trips.

In 1987 K-Tron International designed the K-Tron Institute of Feeder Technology as a separate training division of the company. The Institute provides technical training for customers and employees and is responsible for administering staff development programs at the Pitman site. Incorporated into a "Wellness Program" designed by the Human Resources Dept. and offered through the Institute, are courses offered free of charge to employees on CPR, Back Injury Prevention, and Handling Hazardous Materials. Free screenings for cholesterol are being arranged in cooperation with the American Health Foundation and physical fitness awareness is being promoted through monthly company newsletters and issuance of "Health Passports," a personal record-keeping booklet for charting nutritional and medical information. Company-subsidized health club memberships are being considered and on-site aerobics classes are conducted by and for employees. K-Tron Corporation also sponsors a company softball team and company golf tournaments and ski outings.

K-Tron International, Inc. is committed to promoting wellness through physical fitness programs, education and training while emphasizing that the responsibility for long-term health and longevity is primarily an individual responsibility.

KELLOGG COMPANY

Kellogg Company is a diversified international company specializing in the manufacture and marketing of quality convenience foods. The Company's product base features ready-to-eat cereals,

---

Reprinted courtesy of Kellogg Company.

frozen pies and waffles, toaster pastries, soups and soup bases, yogurt and snack items. While Kellogg's® is recognized worldwide as the leading brand in ready-to-eat cereals, other well-known company brands include Mrs. Smith's®, Eggo®, LeGout®, Whitney's®, and Shirriff®.

Kellogg products are manufactured in 17 countries and distributed in 130 countries around the world. More than 17,000 people are employed by Kellogg Company in manufacturing, distribution, and management.

At Kellogg Company, interest in nutrition, health, and quality is nothing new. The very reason the company was founded in 1906 was to manufacture and sell grain-based food products that were nutritious, tasty alternatives to the heavy, fat-laden meals of the pre-World War I era.

Eighty years later, many science-based groups are recommending that consumers increase the amounts of whole grains, fruits, and vegetables in their diets, and reduce their consumption of fats. More and more consumers are recognizing the importance of proper diet in supporting active lifestyles and promoting wellness and longevity. Through various media, Kellogg disseminates important health and nutrition information, including the distribution of consumer publications.

Most recently, the Company distributed, in cereal packages, over 12 million copies of Health Passport, an educational booklet published by the American Health Foundation. The 15-page publication provides suggested guidelines for healthy lifestyles.

The Company's commitment to health, education and fitness is further evidenced by programs developed for employees. Living healthy and long is the focus of Kellogg Company's "Feeling Gr-r-reat"℠ Employee Health and Fitness Program which is designed to create awareness of healthy lifestyles and motivate employees to make positive lifestyle changes.

Kellogg's Feeling Gr-r-reat Program is unique from many other corporate programs in several ways.

First, the Company provides all employees, hourly and salaried, with an opportunity to participate in the program.

Second, the Company supports its programs with comprehensive health communications targeted to the needs of employees, families and retirees. The Company also publishes materials on a

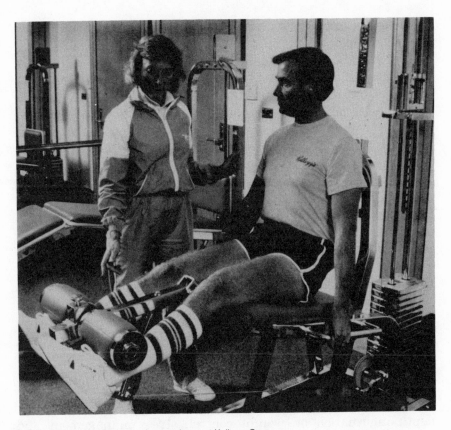

Exercise physiologist instructing employee at Kellogg Company.

regular basis to communicate class schedules, special programs and recognize member achievements.

Finally, due to our broad-based activities and the holistic nature of our health and fitness program, we estimate that 60% of our eligible employees participated in a Feeling Gr-r-reat sponsored program during 1988.

Employees at our Corporate Headquarters and Battle Creek manufacturing facility are able to participate in a regimen of individual or group exercise programs at one of our two on-site fitness centers. The fitness centers are staffed by YMCA professionals having advanced degrees in health-related fields. The centers have single-station, muscle-toning equipment and a variety of aerobics equipment including rowing machines, treadmills, and stationary bicycles selected to exercise all the major muscle groups.

At our other cereal plant locations, where the size of the work force does not make it feasible to build fitness centers, the Company has worked closely with the National YMCA to introduce exercise health programs in cooperation with existing fitness center facilities in the area. Membership at these locations, as is the case with the Battle Creek fitness centers, is funded through a Company subsidy and employee-paid membership fees.

Beyond the fitness centers, a wide variety of health promotion and health education activities support our commitment to a total fitness program. On-site health screening, blood pressure readings and cholesterol checks are several of the many programs made available to employees to heighten their health awareness.

Educational mini-seminars are available in Battle Creek each month. A videotape is made of each program for individuals unable to attend during scheduled times, or for those who want to share the information with their families. Topics addressed include a variety of medical issues—cancer (skin, prostate, breast, uterine and colorectal), PMS, osteoporosis, cholesterol and diet, stress management, and others.

Additionally, health promotion programs, which meet once each week for a period of eight to ten weeks, provide greater in-depth information on weight control, stress management and smoking cessation.

A health promotion program is not complete without a mental well-being component. The Employee Assistance Program is a confidential diagnostic and referral service to help resolve personal problems or concerns. Assessment, counseling and referral services are available to all employees, dependents, and retirees at no cost. Concerns commonly dealt with include: marital and family relationships, finances, substance abuse, dependent care, legal issues, and any other concerns that might have an impact on an individual's mental wellness.

W. K. Kellogg, founder of Kellogg Company, devoted much of his personal time toward the "promotion of the health, education, and welfare of mankind." The Feeling Gr-r-reat Program is only one example of how Kellogg Company continues to put into practice our founder's commitment to healthy lifestyles. Consistent with Mr. Kellogg's commitment, the theme of our Feeling Gr-r-reat Program is to "Live as well as you can, as long as you can."

KEMPER NATIONAL P&C COMPANIES

The Kemper National P&C Companies, members of the Kemper Group, write most types of property and casualty insurance throughout the U.S. and in some foreign markets. Headquartered in Long Grove, Illinois, the companies have the 17th largest property-casualty operations in the U.S. and employ about 9,600 people.

Kemper's overall commitment to employee wellness includes company-sponsored diet, stop-smoking and breast self-exam workshops as well as cardiac risk and blood pressure screenings. The company headquarters offers aerobics classes on premises, a 1.5-mile Parcourse Fitness Circuit on the grounds and employee discounts for the Kemper Lakes 18-hole championship golf course and tennis club. The five interconnecting lakes that surround the home office are open free-of-charge to employees and their families for small boats and fishing. The company also provides information and support for those employees providing care for older adults.

Kemper helps its employees' general well-being through its award-winning employee assistance program, one of the first of its kind which has served as a model for others. The Personal Assistance Program was pioneered in 1962 to assist employees with alcohol problems by former chairman of the board James S. Kemper, Jr., himself a recovering alcoholic who saw first-hand the toll that alcoholism can take on individuals, their employers and families.

The program has since expanded to cover a wide range of living problems affecting job performance, such as drug addiction,

---

Reprinted courtesy of Kemper National P&C Companies.

family and interpersonal relationships, illness, physical handicaps and compulsive behavior. Says program manager Mary Ellen Kane, "We counsel employees on everything from adolescent problems to aging."

The counselors have helped more than 4,400 people since 1974, when statistics were first kept, or an average of 374 employees a year. Additionally, program staff have consulted with more than 3,300 managers and supervisors to help them resolve employee job problems.

The program reports a recovery rate of about 70 percent for alcoholics and 80 percent for people with other types of living problems.

Kane became familiar with the program after seeking counseling herself. She is assisted by two full-time counselors in the headquarters and nurses in three of the larger offices who receive special training in alcoholism and family counseling.

Depending on the employee and the problem, counselors hold one or more sessions by phone or in person and may refer the employee to a mental health clinic or professional, treatment center or self-help group.

Says Kemper Chief Executive Officer Joseph E. Luecke, "Helping our employees deal with problems in their lives is not only the proper thing to do, it's a good bottom-line investment. As I see it, we have three choices when personal problems interfere with an employee's performance over a period of time: We can put up with the inefficiency and the poor company image projected, which costs money; we can fire the employee and hire and train a replacement, which costs money; or we can help the person deal with the problem, which benefits us both."

Statistics bear this out. Kemper research shows that employees with living problems cost the company about 25 percent of their annual salary in lost productivity and errors. Over a twelve-year period, 25 percent of the salaries of those in the program totaled $13.6 million. Compare that to the $1.6 million cost of the program over the 12-year period and you have better than an eight-to-one cost benefit ratio.

But according to program manager Kane, it's the stories behind the numbers that make the program worthwhile.

Says one Kemper employee and former cocaine abuser, "Through the Personal Assistance Program, I was referred to Cocaine Anonymous, Alcoholics Anonymous and Narcotics Anonymous. By participating in these programs, I realized that people do care. I started to develop self-esteem and to take charge of my life. Thanks to the program I can now deal with reality."

Another employee came to treatment drinking more than a quart of scotch every day. The counselor arranged hospitalization in an alcoholic treatment center. The man arrived drunk for his 28-day stay after consuming two fifths of scotch and a half-dozen Librium capsules. He later became a Kemper executive and hasn't had a drink since.

Says CEO Luecke, "Employees have told us they joined Kemper because any company with such an enlightened approach to employee relations is the kind of company they want to work for. We price ourselves in that reputation and take that commitment seriously."

KIMBERLY-CLARK CORPORATION

Kimberly-Clark Corporation, its consolidated subsidiaries and equity companies, are engaged in a worldwide business employing advanced technologies in absorbency, fiber-forming, and other fields. The Corporation's world headquarters is located in Dallas, Texas, and operating units are managed from operations headquarters in Neenah, Wisconsin, and Roswell, Georgia.

Kimberly-Clark Corporation, founded over 100 years ago, manufactures and markets a wide range of products (most of which are made from natural and synthetic fibers) for personal care, health care, and other uses in the home, business, and industry. The Corporation also produces and markets specialty papers requiring specialized technology in development or application, as well as traditional paper and related products for newspaper publishing and other communication needs.

In addition to manufacturing operations, the company has a transportation sector including: a commercial airline, Midwest Express Airlines; a machinery design, fabrication and installa-

Reprinted courtesy of Kimberly-Clark Corporation.

tion organization; and an aviation maintenance, service, and refurbishing business.

Kimberly-Clark recognizes employee health as a priority, and in 1977 developed the Health Management Program, a comprehensive worksite health promotion program. The program objectives include: (1) to achieve a higher level of wellness and productivity in employees, (2) to reduce absenteeism, and (3) to reduce the rate of escalating health care costs. The program strives to improve health and prevent illness by providing a number of voluntary employee services, including medical screening, exercise stress testing, health risk management (e.g., exercise prescription, back injury prevention programs, cardiac rehabilitation, and cholesterol education programs), an Employee Assistance Program, Occupational Health Nursing services, and limited primary care. The Corporation believes in disease prevention and early intervention. The rate of increase in health care costs can be reduced by helping employees take responsibility for their own health and safety.

The Health Management Program in Neenah is located in the Health Services Center, which includes an 8,000-square-foot multiphasic screening unit and a 37,000-square-foot Exercise Facility with an indoor running track, an Olympic-size pool, weight and equipment room, saunas, whirlpool, and locker facilities. In addition, a 2.0-mile outdoor walking/running trail is available. The program provides services to over 7,000 salaried and hourly employees, retirees, and spouses.

The health team members includes two physicians, Employee Assistance Program professionals, Occupational Health Nurses, Family Nurse Practitioners, technicians, health and fitness specialists, lifeguards, and clerical assistants.

The Health Management Program was expanded to the Roswell, Georgia operations headquarters with annual health screenings performed since 1981 and a complete Health Management Program and Facility in 1986. This Health Center includes a 3,000-square-foot multiphasic screening unit and a 21,000-square-foot Exercise Facility with an outdoor running trail, Olympic-size pool, weight and exercise classroom, saunas, whirlpool, and locker facilities. Over 1,100 employees, retirees, and spouses have access to health promotion services at the facility.

The Corporation offers health screening and exercise facility services to both salaried and hourly employees and retirees. In January of 1982 the program was made available to spouses of employees and retirees. Employees and retirees participate in the program at no charge. Spouses are charged a nominal fee to cover health screening costs.

A health screening is required before participating in the exercise program. The screening program consists of a health risk appraisal, a blood chemistry panel including lipid studies, multiphasic screening tests, a complete physical examination, and exercise testing by treadmill or bicycle ergometer. At the completion of the screening, participants have an "exit interview"—referred to by the staff as "the teachable moment." Data are evaluated and a "wellness prescription" is established by the physician, nurse practitioner, health and fitness specialist, or Occupational Health Nurse. The wellness prescription outlines as exercise program and may also recommend follow-up by the in-house Employee Assistance Program, the employee's Occupational Health Nurse, or referral to his or her personal physician for further evaluation or treatment. Screening also enables the health professionals to reinforce already existing positive lifestyle habits and attitudes.

Emphasis is also placed on special health promotion projects. Since 1982, Kimberly-Clark has participated in National High Blood Pressure Month activities. The hypertension screening and tracking program is tailored by Occupational Health Nurses to the specific needs of the employee population at each Kimberly-Clark location in the United States and Canada. Blood pressure tracking is performed on a continual basis for employees with elevated readings. Other activities to promote employee health and safety include: a Healthy Back Program, a Cholesterol Education Program, including assistance with menu evaluation for cafeteria foods, and health presentations.

Occupational Health Nurses (OHN's) provide nursing services to employees at 32 Kimberly-Clark locations in the United States. The goal of OHN services is to deliver a comprehensive health service to employees at the worksite, focusing on health promotion, health maintenance, and injury prevention. While the administration of on-site first aid is still an important function, the emphasis is on medical surveillance, physical assessment, and health promotion. The OHN functions as a gatekeeper for entry into the health care delivery system within Kimberly-Clark and the community, and is increasingly involved in counseling employees to become wise purchasers of health care and to enter the appropriate level of the health care delivery system.

The Employee Assistance Program provides professional, confidential services to employees with special personal health problems which interfere with their job performance. These problems include alcohol or other drug abuse, mental health problems, family or marital conflict, and financial or legal difficulties. Program services are available to employees, their families and retirees and include problem identification, short-term motivational counseling, referral to community treatment resources, and follow-up to ensure that results are achieved. Strict confidentiality is critical to the success of this program.

The goal of Kimberly-Clark's Health Management Program is to contribute to the Corporation's climate of care and concern for its employees by helping Kimberly-Clark people in all locations achieve better health. Well-informed, healthy employees are happier, safer, more productive, have less absenteeism, and are more likely to have lower health care costs. Through accessible and cost-effective health screening, limited primary care, exercise programs, nursing services, and an Employee Assistance Program, an individual's level of health can be improved. WE AIM TO BE THE BEST AT CARING summarizes the health team's goal in meeting the needs of Kimberly-Clark people.

L. L. BEAN, INC.

L. L. Bean, Inc. sells quality apparel, footwear, and equipment directly to outdoor-oriented Americans. In 1988, 76 years after its founding, the company reached nearly half a billion dollars in sales. Located in Freeport, Maine, we do more than 87 percent of our business by catalog. Employment is approximately 3,000 year

---

Reprinted courtesy of L. L. Bean, Inc.

round, with an additional 2,000 seasonal employees hired for the peak as Christmas approaches.

Leon Leonwood Bean founded the mail order business in 1912 with this simple philosophy: "Sell good merchandise at a reasonable profit, treat your customers like human beings and they'll always come back for more." The company calls this creed "L. L.'s" golden rule and adherence to it has made L. L. Bean, Inc. successful.

Most of this success stems from the performance of our employees. The company's president, Leon Gorman, "L. L.'s" grandson, firmly believes that it is the individual performance of each employee that makes a successful company.

"Performance through people" summarizes our outlook and in Leon's words, "People with ability, given an opportunity to perform in a motivating environment, will achieve the 'best' performance." This ability includes a physical dimension and a mental one.

From a small beginning in 1982, L. L. Bean's Health and Fitness Program has contributed to the company's prosperity. Our employees have made the program part of their workday lives. At the same time the health and fitness programs help employees in their efforts to attain improved health and well-being for themselves and their families.

Many employees at L. L. Bean enjoy the outdoors, and the formal program helps optimize that enthusiasm while involving more people. When an addition to the main offices was built in 1982, Leon included a fully equipped exercise room just because he felt it was the right thing to do. A part-time consultant taught classes while developing activities. The program continues to grow because of Leon's increasing commitment to fitness and his realization that healthy and fit employees will be more productive in their personal and company lives.

The Health and Fitness Program was designed to provide all employees with the opportunity to improve their health habits. All L. L. Bean employees, seasonal and retirees included, are encouraged to participate. The company has four fitness rooms at different locations throughout the company. They are open weekdays from 6 A.M. to 6 P.M., with one room having night hours 11 P.M. to 2 A.M. Monday through Friday. A "buddy" system, where two employees can open the other rooms at any time, adds flexibility.

The emphasis of the program, like that of the company's, is on non-competitive, recreational activities that people of varying abilities can pursue during their lifetime. The facilities contain treadmills, bicycles, rowing machines, cross-country ski machines, stair climbers, universal weights, and free weights.

In addition to the fitness rooms, we offer a wide variety of health and fitness classes. The company has concentrated on structured courses over the past few years. Through surveys, course evaluations, and daily communication with employees we have been able to develop programs which meet employee needs. Here are the classes currently being offered.

Activity Classes

Lap Swimming
Adult Swimming Lessons
Cross-country Skiing
Aerobic Exercise
Aerobic Dance
Full-Figured Aerobics
Body Works (Tone and
   Strengthen)
Hiking
Kayaking
Aerobic Cycling
Walking
Jogging
Retiree Exercise
Tennis
Yoga
Ballroom Dance

Health Classes

Smoking Cessation
Heart Club
   (Cholesterol Education)
Stress Management
Weight-Loss Programs
Weigh-ins
First Aid
CPR
Back Schools
Worksite Exercise Programs
Self-Breast Exams

Classes are taught by our fitness staff as well as by other qualified employees and external consultants. The staff consists of a Health and Fitness Specialist who has an M.S. in Exercise Physiology, four Exercise Technicians, each with a B.S. in a Health/Fitness-related field, and a Health and Fitness secretary.

When employees enter the health and fitness programs they receive one and one-half hours of health screening and orientation. Emphasis is on exercising within one's abilities and conditioning level, and on the safe use of equipment. In the past year we have added computerized Health Risk Appraisal and a General Fitness Assessment. These are used to counsel employees on their cardiovascular risk factors and to prescribe individualized exercise programs. Throughout, we discuss individual responsibility for health, and we encourage participants to assume that responsibility.

Individual responsibility for health and safety on and off the job places a concurrent responsibility on the company for health and safety on the job. Recognizing that, the Health and Fitness program is part of the company's overall Employee Health and Safety Program. The Health and Safety Program assigns and promotes safe, consistent employee practices throughout the company. The company currently restricts smoking to only one area in each building. Eventually we would like to be "smoke-free."

For example, we cannot, in good faith, ask employees to stop smoking at home if they are being exposed, unprotected, to fumes or dust at work. We cannot expect them to wear seat belts or follow safety rules off the job if we do not strive to provide a healthy and safe environment on the job. Similarly, the offering of aerobic exercise and stretching programs to office workers cannot be separated from the offering of safe and ergonomically designed workstations.

We are increasing the integration of Health and Fitness with Occupational Health and Safety. The staffs work together in promoting and administering Health Risk Appraisals: In hypertension screening and follow-up, in teaching work station adjustments and exercises to individual departments, in combining "back schools" with health and fitness program classes, and in helping rehabilitate injured workers back into the workforce.

We communicate our programs to the local medical community, and ask for their cooperation in helping to maintain their patients'—our employees'—health and safety. To that end we have given facilities tours to approximately 80 local physicians and other health care providers in the last two to three years, and we ask them to encourage their patients to participate in our program.

We have attained approximately 30–40 percent participation in our health and fitness programs. The easiest employees to reach have been the ones who would be fit regardless of the programs. The hardest for us to reach are the hourly employees in production jobs who leave work tired and have little flexibility in their schedules. We are trying more creative approaches to reach this population and now put more emphasis into outreach activities where we bring the programs to our employees.

As our Health and Fitness program grows we will see it integrate more and more with the mainstream of our business. Like benefits, compensation, and training and development, health and fitness will become an integral part of a business goal: superior performance for L. L. Bean through the superior performance of our employees. The well-being of the company and our employees are inextricably linked.

MANNINGTON MILLS, INC.

Concern for quality permeates every aspect of Mannington Mills, Inc., from the quality of its products to the employees' quality of life. Since it was founded in 1915, the floorcovering manufacturing company has been a family business. Today, the same close-knit family feeling still exists. This history has much to do with the scope of the company's fitness and wellness programs.

Mannington's corporate headquarters, as well as its largest operating subsidiary in employees and earnings—Mannington Resilient Floors—is situated in Salem, N.J. The Salem location covers 328 acres and employs nearly 700 people. It is also the company's site for manufacturing 12-foot-wide sheet vinyl flooring. The sheet vinyl is sold through an international distribution network.

Three other subsidiaries are also part of the company: Wellco Business Carpet in Calhoun, Ga.; Mannington Ceramic Tile in Lexington, N.C.; and Mannington Wood Floors in High Point,

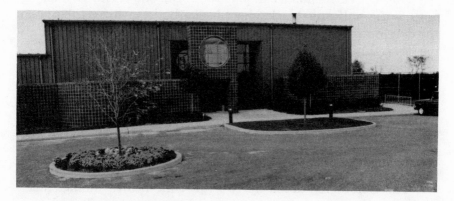

Mannington Mills fitness center at Salem, New Jersey.

N.C. Altogether, the four subsidiaries have more than 1,500 employees.

In 1986, Mannington Mills was named one of the "10 Best Companies to Work For In New Jersey" by the *Business Journal of New Jersey*. The publication said, "What is perhaps most outstanding about Mannington . . . is its $2 million employee fitness center." Built in 1984, the H. Arthur Williams Fitness Center was named in honor of the company president at the time. (He retired in 1987 after 26 years of service.)

John B. Campbell II, Chairman of the Board and grandson of the company's founder, originated the concept of a Mannington Fitness Center. Management's active belief in physical fitness is apparent: most top executives work out on a regular basis and they encourage employees to stay fit, with or without the use of the Fitness Center.

The Fitness Center serves as the nucleus for all health-oriented programs. The two-story structure occupies almost 16,000 square feet of floor space indoors. It was built in the back of Mannington's site, just a minute's ride away from the main building.

Indoor facilities include: coed weight room with 19 Nautilus or Universal machines, free weights, electronic rowing and treadmill machines; regulation-size basketball court; aerobic room; game room with pool table and table tennis; locker rooms with showers, steam room, and whirlpool.

Outdoor enthusiasts can play tennis on one of four courts, jog around the half-mile track, shoot basketballs, or hit golf balls on the driving range. There is also a full-size softball field, although it's located near Mannington's entrance.

Obviously, lack of variety is not a problem. It was important—in creating the Fitness Center—to appeal to the varied tastes of hundreds of employees, spouses, and retirees. It seems the formula is working because the facility boasts an average of 100 users per day. Because many employees are shift workers, the Fitness Center has a daily schedule to accommodate workers of three different shifts.

The Center is staffed by two full-time health management professionals and three part-time aerobic instructors. To add even more youthful enthusiasm, a college intern program was started in 1986. The interns get practical experience as they assist in various activities.

A large amount of time, effort and other resources goes into the planning and implementation of fitness-related programs. Why bother? According to Carl Sempier, former President of Mannington Resilient Floors, there are several good reasons. He says, "Good physical health is fundamental to a sound mental attitude. If people take good care of their bodies, their minds will be in better shape too."

Some activities also promote a feeling of working together, a sense of belonging. Sempier says, "We organize a lot of team sports . . . not only because people enjoy them, but because sports go along with the family spirit we have at Mannington." There are company leagues for softball, tennis, golf, volleyball, pool, table tennis, and basketball.

Another aspect of the Fitness Center is education. "We would rather invest in prevention and help employees avoid certain health problems," says one staff member. The emphasis is on getting people to eliminate unhealthy behaviors and habits.

For example, Mannington holds smoking-cessation classes with the cooperation of a local American Cancer Society chapter. Having the classes gives smokers who are thinking of quitting a little extra motivation and support. One ex-smoker says, "I wanted to quit but didn't think I could do it on my own. The sessions gave me the push I needed. Also, it was a big help talking to people who were going through the same experience."

That philosophy of prevention has inspired a range of events. Past program topics include nutrition, back pain, cardiac-risk reduction, CPR, blood-pressure screening, and health-risk appraisals. Some workshops are targeted specifically to women: breast cancer, pap tests, PMS and menopausal women's health, and stress and the working woman.

For people who want to shed extra pounds, the Fitness Center holds weight loss competitions. The contests inject some fun into a usually dreary undertaking and provide added motivation.

Employees who retire from Mannington are still considered part of the family and they share in the Fitness Center benefits. The company's Retirees Association holds its monthly meetings there. Each month a speaker addresses an issue that is of special concern to senior citizens; examples include: finances on a fixed income, Social Security, blood pressure control, and living with arthritis.

On the other end of the age spectrum, the very young are carefully supervised while parents are working out. This service is provided free of charge. Older children are not neglected either. They are eligible to use all Fitness Center facilities.

Mannington's Fitness Center is a place to work out, shape up, feel good, slim down, play hard, and have fun. It makes Mannington Mills a better place to work and, hopefully, helps members of the Mannington family lead healthier, more productive lives.

MICHIGAN BELL

Michigan Bell provides communication services in 74 counties statewide, serving more than 3 million customers and residents. With more than 17,000 employees, the corporation is one of the state's largest employers. Michigan Bell's state-of-the-art communications network, consisting of advanced digital switches and fiber optic technologies, enables the corporation to offer advanced products and services to customers.

Reprinted courtesy of Michigan Bell.

Although advanced technology is essential to the functioning of the tele-communication industry, our most highly valued asset remains—our employees.

In 1984, the implementation of the Wellness Program was recommended by the Corporate Medical Director to the Officers. The Officers approved the concept and provided funds to develop a Corporate Wellness Program. The primary goal of the program is:

> To assist employees in maintaining and/or improving their general sense of well-being, energy levels and overall quality of life through various activities designed to increase knowledge of and establish positive attitudes about personal wellness.

The Program is implemented on three levels: awareness, programs, and a supportive environment (Figure 1).

AWARENESS

Health Risk Appraisal. Developing a sense of awareness concerning wellness among the employee population was an essential first step. In 1984, a Health Risk Appraisal (HRA) developed by the University of Michigan Fitness Research Center, consultants to the program, was administered. Both corporate and union officials encouraged employees to participate in this project. Participants received personalized feedback from the university, and the corporation received aggregate data which served as a needs assessment. Currently, the HRA process is being repeated to determine the present status of the employee population, and their feelings and concerns about the Wellness Program.

Communication. A variety of communication ideas have been used to bring the Wellness Program to the attention of employees. In-house forums, Wellness program schedules, and a purchased communication program have been used to bring regular information to employees about various health and wellness issues. The Wellness logo has been used frequently and serves as a recognized symbol of the program.

PROGRAMS

Based on employee needs identified by the HRA, a variety of programs are available to all employees—management and non-management. It is not uncommon to find non-management and upper-management employees in the same classes. Examples of programs include: weight reduction, smoking cessation, healthy back, various levels of exercise, walking, stress management, breast self-examination, and blood pressure and cholesterol screening. All programs are offered statewide—they're not limited to corporate headquarters or a large metropolitan area. Participation in all programs is voluntary.

Some of the programs are implemented with the help of other corporate groups. Together, the Corporate Education Center and Employee Assistance Program developed and implemented the stress management program. The Nursing staff has presented breast self-examination programs, and blood pressure and cholesterol education and screening programs to thousands of employees throughout Michigan. And, the Healthy Back video and program were developed with the cooperative efforts of the Safety department, the Audio-Visual department, and two non-corporate organizations. In some programs, employees are required to make a monetary commitment when participating; however, the corporation does subsidize all programs.

The Walking Program is probably the most successful program with more than 2,000 employees registered. Interest in this program was generated by employees who wanted to walk on their lunch breaks. Currently, twenty-eight measured-mile maps are available for walking routes adjacent to work location areas throughout the state. This is the only program that offers incentive awards, which are given to employees when they walk various mileage increments. The most promising facts about this program, which probably contributes to its success, include: employees wanted it, it is inexpensive to administer, it seems to attract office/clerical personnel who have very little physical activities during work hours, it improves cardiovascular functioning, a high risk factor, and is considered to be a safe activity for most groups of people. In fact it is probably attracting the segment of our population we should be most concerned about—inactive persons.

SUPPORTIVE ENVIRONMENT

A supportive environment completes and complements the implementation of Wellness at Michigan Bell. Figure 1 lists examples of environmental support mechanisms. A full-time Wellness Coordinator, who is a masters prepared nurse certified in Occupational Health, administers the program.

Encouraging management, non-management and Quality of Work Life groups to input into the development of the program sets a tone of cooperation and support which enhances the concept of wellness. A company-wide policy to create a smoke-free environment went into effect July 1, 1987. Flextime allows employees to manage their work and personal lives more effectively. An employee fitness center was opened in the headquarters complex, and plans for five more in other Michigan Bell buildings have been developed. Fitness Center equipment includes treadmills, bikes, mats, seven pieces of resistance-type equipment, and aerobic workout space. Locker and shower areas are adjacent to the workout area. Registered employees are able to use the center seven days a week from 6:00 A.M. to 11:00 P.M. There are no registration fees.

Although the implementation model is divided into three levels, in reality no boundaries exist since all levels rely on the others for the planning and implementation of the Wellness Program. The program is dynamic and evolving as new ideas, stresses, and information necessitate change. Change is an essential characteristic of our program, since the corporation, telecommunications industry and the employees, both in their personal and work lives are constantly experiencing change.

The Michigan Bell Wellness Program's primary goal is to assist employees in maintaining and/or improving their general sense of well-being and overall quality of life. By creating a work environment supportive of positive health practices it is hoped that costs associated with insurance claims, sick leaves and/or disability will be impacted resulting in an improved quality of work life environment. Such an environment will enhance the attainment of corporate goals.

FIGURE 1

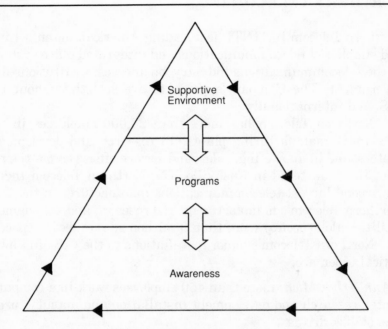

Supportive Environment:	Supportive Top Management
	Budget
	Staff
	Management participation
	Employee participation
	Quality of Worklife groups
	Flextime
	Smoking Policy
	Corporate Sports Battle
	Fitness Centers
Programs:	Weight Watchers at Work
	Smoking Cessation
	Healthy Back
	Exercise classes
	Walking Program
	Stress Management
	Breast Self-Exam Programs
	Blood Pressure & Cholesterol Research Study
Awareness:	Health Risk Appraisal
	Screening Programs
	In-house Newsletters: TIE LINES & UPDATE
	Monthly Communication Program: Posters & Flyers
	Wellness schedules

NORTHERN TELECOM INC.

Northern Telecom Inc. (NTI) is a leading American manufacturer and supplier of telecommunications and integrated office systems to the telecommunications industry, businesses, institutions and government. The Company's products are sold throughout the U.S. and internationally.

Northern Telecom has more than 20,000 employees in the U.S. in 11 manufacturing plants, 13 research and development centers, and in marketing, sales, and service offices across the nation. Headquartered in Nashville, TN, Northern Telecom Inc. is the second largest telecommunications manufacturer in the U.S. Northern Telecom's manufacturing and research and development facilities alone occupy more than 3 million square feet of space.

Northern Telecom's major installations in the U.S., in alphabetical order, are:

• *Ann Arbor, Mich:* more than 450 employees work in a computer center, research and development installation and manufacture a line of disk drives.
• *Atlanta, GA:* about 1,300 employees manufacture and market digital transmission equipment.
• *Dallas, TX:* about 2,000 employees work in the marketing and support of private branch exchanges and digital switching equipment, and research and development.
• *Morton Grove, Ill.:* about 850 employees manufacture the supporting hardware used by telephone companies to interconnect their central switching centers to home and business locations.
• *Raleigh/Durham/RTP, NC:* four manufacturing plants employ more than 6,000 employees manufacturing digital central office switching equipment for telephone companies and switches for interexchange carriers.
• *Santa Clara, CA:* about 1,200 employees manufacture digital business communications systems or private branch exchanges.

• *San Diego, CA:* about 350 employees design and manufacture semiconductor components in the company's integrated circuit plant.
• *West Palm Beach, FL:* 600 employees manufacture printed circuit boards and hybrid substrates.

Northern Telecom is unique in its approach to employee health, wellness and fitness. We employ 29 health professionals (primarily registered professional nurses) in 20 Health Centers across the United States. The health professionals are responsible for coordinating all aspects of employee health care, from traditional "illness and injury care" to health education and counseling and fitness programs.

We consider fitness programs to be one small component of an overall health and wellness program called the Northern Telecom Health Enhancement Program (HEP). This program is marketed to employees using the "brand logo" Invest in Yourself. Under that theme, we are encouraging employees to take charge of their health and participate in one or more of our HEP activities.

Our major programs are offered on a nationwide basis to all employees. Currently, the major Health Enhancement Programs are:

• *Health Check:* This is the "flagship" of all HEP programs. Health Check measures health risks by completion of a Health Risk Appraisal; measurements of blood pressure, total cholesterol and HDL cholesterol, percent body fat, total body strength and flexibility and cardiac fitness as measured by a 6 minute submaximal stationary bicycle test. The results of Health Check allow an employee to see what health risks they have and then use one or more of the following programs to work on specific risk areas.
• *High Blood Pressure Control:* This program encourages employees to learn about their blood pressure, know what their own pressure is and act to control it if it is elevated. NTI health professionals work with employees' personal physicians to help monitor blood pressure problems and progress.

• *Cholesterol Control Program:* Designed to cope with one of the largest risk factors for heart disease, this program allows measurement of blood cholesterol from a simple fingerstick with results in 3 minutes. Follow-up counseling focuses on diet, exercise and stress reduction.

• *Weight Management:* Different NTI locations offer a variety of programs in weight management. We have a general commitment to always discuss the role of exercise in weight control. An emphasis is also placed on percent body fat vs. weight alone.

• *Fitness Challenge:* A 12-week program designed to start at whatever fitness level the individual is at currently and, through planned aerobic activities, increase that level over a 12-week period. Some of our locations have completely outfitted fitness centers with muscle toning/building equipment, cardiovascular equipment and aerobics classes.

• *Stress Management:* NTI is a high-change, high-stress environment. We are attempting to reach our employees with innovative programs to help manage their stress. Stress management is also included in all management training courses.

• *Employee Assistance Programs (EAP):* We consider EAP to be part of our preventive wellness strategy. EAPs are there to provide confidential counseling in the areas of marital/family, financial, legal, alcohol/drug and other personal problems. EAP counselors often refer employees into one or more of the existing HEP programs.

• *Smoking Cessation:* A very important program as we move closer to a smokefree workplace. We offer a variety of classes both on-site and partial reimbursement for approved off-site programs.

Summary: In addition to the specific programs listed, we offer a vast variety of shorter programs throughout the year. Some are offered as "brown bag lunches" or "lunch n' learns," others are presented at employee quality circles or at management meetings. We use a multitude of approaches to deliver our products.

At Northern Telecom, we view fitness as one small component of a total health enhancement perspective. We do believe that it is a very important component but it should not be the total focus of wellness programs. We fulfill our commitment to our people by providing them quality programs run by highly qualified health professionals. Nearly 50% of our nurses have their Master's degree in their health specialty. Having an on-site staff of this quality allows us to offer what we believe are some of the best health programs available to employees anywhere.

NORTHWESTERN NATIONAL LIFE INSURANCE COMPANY

The NWNL Companies, Inc. is a diversified insurance company based in Minneapolis. It is among the 50 largest life insurance companies in the U.S., with $77 billion of insurance in force and consolidated assets of $7.5 billion. It employs approximately 2,500 people.

Health and well-being play a crucial role in the life and health insurance business and NWNL has a natural interest in promoting them. When the concept of wellness in the workplace started gaining popularity in the early 1980s, NWNL began examining existing wellness programs based upon two objectives. The first was to sponsor a wellness program for its own employees. The second was to offer group insurance buyers a wellness program as a supplement to their insurance and employee benefits package.

NWNL chose one program that met both needs. It was Staywell, a program developed and marketed by Control Data Corporation. Staywell was introduced at NWNL in 1982. It was available to all full-time employees with more than two years of service at a cost to each participant of $24 per year.

The Staywell program had two key components. The first was health screening, which included a detailed questionnaire covering each participant's health and lifestyle, a fitness assessment, and a blood sample. This information was analyzed by computer and developed into a health risk profile with detailed information about each person's physical condition.

The other major component of the program was the action phase. Depending on the results of the health risk profile, employ-

---

Reprinted courtesy of Northwestern National Life Insurance Co.

ees could participate in lifestyle change courses that addressed issues such as weight loss, smoking cessation, relaxation, nutrition, fitness, and blood pressure.

As the wellness program became more firmly established, NWNL's Staywell Task Force developed formal goals and objectives that were announced in 1984. The two overall goals were: (1) To express the company's care and concern for the well-being of all employees of the NWNL family of companies by promoting good health and mental well-being; and (2) To pioneer and model to the community, the industry and to its clients its commitment to good health.

NWNL sponsored Staywell for three years and the program enjoyed considerable popularity and participation. In 1984, the company opened participation to more employees, making it available to all employees regardless of length of service and eliminating all employee costs. NWNL also provided 50% of the time for wellness-related activities, which had previously been conducted solely on employees' personal time.

In 1985, the company decided to launch its own wellness program, one more closely tailored to the specific needs and interests of NWNL employees. The major changes were: (1) greater emphasis on on-site exercise classes and facilities, and (2) a wider variety of one-time seminars as opposed to longer courses on more general topics.

Employee interest is the key to NWNL's wellness program, and it has resulted in a comprehensive range of activities. The major components of the program include:

Annual Fitness Assessment. Each year, employees may participate at no cost in a fitness assessment conducted by the wellness director, a certified specialist. It measures such factors as height and weight, body composition, blood pressure, cardiovascular endurance, muscular strength and flexibility. Participants receive a detailed description of their personal results and suggestions on ways to improve their overall level of fitness. In 1987, 162 employees took part in the assessment.

On-site Exercise Facilities. Two buildings of NWNL's three-building home office complex are equipped with exercise rooms and locker facilities. One room contains a variety of muscle-toning equipment such as a Universal gym, stationary bikes, rowing machine, free weights, arm and leg pulley machine, slant-boards, rebounder, and a VCR with exercise tapes.

The other room is specially designed for aerobics. It features a state-of-the-art neo-shock floor, a built-in sound system, a raised instructor platform and mirrored walls.

Exercise Classes. Each week, NWNL offers 20 hours of fitness classes of varying degrees of intensity. Classes include high-impact aerobics, low-impact aerobics, muscle toning, and pre- and post-natal fitness. They are offered before work, during lunch and after work. Classes are taught by the wellness program director and by contracted professional instructors from a Twin Cities fitness organization. In 1987, 1,046 employees participated.

Exercise class participants pay a fee that covers part of the cost and the company subsidizes the rest. NWNL also gives employees 30 minutes in addition to their 45-minute lunch break to participate in wellness activities, subject to supervisor approval.

"Brown-bag" Wellness Seminars. Approximately once a month, NWNL offers "brown bag seminars" at noon at no cost to employees. Topics during the past year have included employee burnout, PMS, back health, breast health, athletic injury prevention, and food sensitivity and allergies. These seminars are conducted by local experts. Employees may take 30 extra minutes in addition to their lunch break to attend. In 1987, there were 21 seminars, which drew a total of 586 attendees. In addition, the company offered a four-week stress-management course, four-week separate weight-training clinics for men and women, and a six-week "walking to wellness" class.

Weight Watchers. NWNL sponsors Weight Watchers at Work, a specially designed weight-loss program for the needs of working people. It meets once a week over the lunch hour. Participants pay part of the cost and the company subsidizes the remainder. Six hundred participants lost a total of 2,352 pounds in 1987.

Smoke-free Environment. Since January 1, 1986, NWNL has had a smoke-free environment. Smoking is permitted only in very limited areas of two cafeterias. To help employees interested in breaking their smoking habit, NWNL pays part of the cost for smoking cessation classes at work and covers 80% of the cost of any similar classes that employees take after work. In 1987, 18 employees took advantage of the offer. In 1986, 150 took company-sponsored smoking cessation classes, which accounted for most of those who planned to quit.

Other Programs. Throughout the year, NWNL sponsors a variety of other health-related activities. During National Blood Pressure Month, it offers free blood pressure tests to all employees, and 784 took the test in 1987. It offers CPR training and breast health seminars during Cancer Month. In 1988, 307 employees took part in a cholesterol screening and educational seminars to interpret results.

In 1987, NWNL developed a formal written policy on AIDS and sponsored an AIDS education seminar that was attended by 750 employees. According to the 1987 AIDS survey by the Alexander & Alexander Consulting Group, only 19.6% of responding businesses offer AIDS education to employees and only 8.3% have a formal AIDS policy.

Participation statistics demonstrate the popularity of NWNL's wellness program. In 1985, 653 employees participated in Staywell activities. In 1986 the number of wellness participants more than quadrupled, rising to 2,581. In comparison, costs did not even double during that same period. Participation rose even more notably in 1987, when 4,200 took part in wellness activities. (Note: If one employee takes part in seven different activities, he or she will appear on the records as seven participants.)

Statistical measurements of the improvements achieved through wellness are difficult to make because behavioral changes can be attributed to a variety of factors. However, NWNL feels so confident about the effectiveness of its wellness program that it does not feel that an exhaustive cost/benefit study is necessary. The interest and enthusiasm that employees continue to show in company-sponsored activities are sufficient proof that the wellness program is providing valuable benefits.

OHIO BELL

Ohio Bell is a telecommunications company which primarily provides business and residence telephone services to all major cities in the state of Ohio, with the exception of Cincinnati. We currently have 13,600 employees. The Company has supported and provided financial assistance to traditional recreational and individual sports for many years. These, as one might imagine, include softball, basketball, bowling, golf and other activities which our employees are involved in on an after-hours basis.

Because of the developing national interest in physical fitness and wellness, we have arranged to offer many programs and services to our employees in conjunction with those offered by local community organizations. Adjacent to our corporate headquarters in Cleveland there is a fully staffed and equipped fitness center managed by the Cleveland YMCA. This facility offers varied activities supervised by trained personnel and is open during hours convenient to our participants. We inform our employees of available fitness facilities in other communities. For example, in Columbus, we are assisting a local hospital in developing a walking program and establishing fitness objectives for employees to pursue during lunch hours and after work. We have negotiated substantial discounts in membership fees for our employees at this facility and others throughout the state. Corporate discount rates are published through articles in-house and in other company publications.

The possibility of locating exercise centers on Company premises has been evaluated. In addition to diminished floor space there is the additional expense of providing locker room and shower facilities. Qualified trained personnel would be required to operate the facility and the Company is faced with possible liability from any accidents that occur.

Corporately, we have concluded in-house fitness facilities are not feasible at this time because: the difficulty of providing equal

Reprinted courtesy of Ohio Bell. Prepared by Walton R. Garner, M.D., Director, Department of Health, Safety, and Environment, Deoniece Arnold, R.N., B.A., Corporate Nurse, and Russell T. Natoce, District Manager, Benefit Planning and Development.

facilities at each of more than 300 locations; the availability of numerous adequate facilities located in the community and the accessibility of walking programs which require no special facilities or high level training. Additionally, there is a lack of voiced demand for such facilities by the majority of our employees.

Tests were conducted in 1984 and 1985 with a group of Cleveland employees to determine if those who agreed to participate in an Exercise Program, partly supported by the Company, would continue with exercise programs on their own, once the initial program was completed. That study revealed that people will continue with exercise programs only if they have the desire, regardless of the health or financial benefits received from the activity. The number from the test group who continued to participate in exercise programs was very low.

Some clarification may be required as to what a "Wellness" versus a "Fitness" Program is. We feel a good program includes aspects of both.

Our Wellness Programs include:

House Organ Stories and Articles
Health and Safety Publications
Health Risk Appraisals
Nutrition Clinics
Weight Reduction Groups
Breast Self-Examination
Hypertension Testing
Smoking Cessation Clinics
Colds and Flu
AIDS Education and Information
Blood Pressure/Pulse Rate Testing
BP Machines and Weight Scales in lunch room area

Employee Assistance Programs:

Drug/substance abuse and behavioral issues
No Laughing Matter
Stress and Your Health

Family Hope
Soft is the Heart of a Child
Living Through Grief
Know Your Limit
Drugs and the Workplace
Your Wellness Checklist
Supervisor/Steward Training
Alcohol and Your Health
Getting Through The Holidays

Our Medical Department and its Health, Safety and Environment District have designed educational programs to help Ohio Bell employees develop positive attitudes and behaviors which reflect a "healthy lifestyle." Topics are based upon criteria generally recommended by universally accepted fitness programs coupled with individual preferences and disability indicators. Our programs include slide presentations and videotapes relative to the subject. The Wellness Programs are coordinated and presented by all of our Health Consultants (Nurses) throughout the state, ensuring a consistency of the "message delivered." Programs are offered monthly or on special requests from specific work groups. This special scheduling gives departments the flexibility to meet the needs of varied work schedules and alternate shifts while continuing to conduct daily business without disruption.

Health Consultants do not function as mere "band aid" nurses but manage disability programs, operate clinical facilities and instruct employees in the total wellness concept. These personal presentations give our nurses an opportunity to interface with groups of employees throughout the state. We consider the face-to-face contact with our employees to be a vital function and a means of convincing employees that Ohio Bell management truly "cares." Our programs are unique in concept and delivery, as we strive to be concise but thorough in all aspects.

Our first major health program "A Smoke Free Environment" was started in November, 1984. A Smoke-Free Workplace Planning Committee (consisting of managers, union, smokers and non-smokers, men and women) was formed to develop policy recommendations. They assessed the degree of the problem, addressed the assertiveness of non-smokers and evaluated growing awareness associated with this health issue.

A Health Consultant (Nurse) with the assistance of the American Lung Association trained employees to be "Freedom from Smoking" facilitators. These clinics were initially held after-hours, but as part of our continuing effort to move toward a smoke-free environment, we began to offer additional clinics on company time. To enhance the concept of "commitment through ownership," employees paid $50 for participation in the clinic. Total cost was reimbursed if the employee remained smoke-free after one year. Ohio Bell will become a totally smoke-free workplace (except for clearly identified designated smoking areas) on August 8, 1988.

Another unique program is Hypertension. We have trained employees in specific work groups to perform blood pressure testing according to High Blood Pressure Coalition standards. Our Health Consultants supervise procedures when such readings are taken. This approach has helped to eliminate employees fears concerning the usage of "health appraisal information."

The Communication Workers of America (CWA), our union, is regularly consulted when planning special presentations on vital issues such as Drug/Substance Abuse and AIDS. The success of our Employee Assistance Program is largely due to its training of CWA union coordinators and the close, and constant communication with the EAP manager, counselors and psychologists. The EAP is implemented with a broad unified approach. The union-management EAP team reviews policy, gives EAP training and participates in the interviews and interventions with employees.[1]

We, at Ohio Bell feel that active Health and Wellness Programs are essential to provide each employee an opportunity to increase his or her knowledge of the factors that can contribute to a healthier lifestyle and greater personal productivity. Additionally, we are committed to having the best educated, most informed and physically healthy employees of any corporation.

Our Health and Wellness programs help those in our corporate family to understand that Ohio Bell hopes to provide a healthy, considerate work environment with emphasis on the well being of every member of our work force.

Additional benefits to the company will accrue through increased employee productivity, individual self-awareness and diminished health insurance costs.

Ohio Bell considers the Health and Wellness of its people to be paramount in operation of a successful enterprise.

ENDNOTE

1. "EAP Rate Is a Good Investment," *Mid-American Outlook*, Vol. X, No. 4, Ameritrust, Winter 1988.

PACIFIC TELESIS

The Pacific Telesis Group consists of thirteen subsidiary companies, the largest being Pacific Bell. Pacific Bell provides intrastate telecommunications services to most regions of California. Services performed by other subsidiary companies include publishing, international operations, paging and mobile service.

Pacific Bell's administrative center is located in San Ramon, east of San Francisco. The company employs approximately 62,500 employees statewide at several hundred locations which vary in employee count from 1 to 7,000.

Pacific Bell has a department of Health Services which provides health risk assessments, health promotions, and disease prevention activities as its major clinical function.

Formulation of a corporate wellness strategy for Pacific Bell began in 1982. Currently, the Health Services Department offers employees a range of activities for primary and secondary disease prevention. The wellness programs support the corporate goal of health care cost containment by preventing disease, promoting good health, and enhancing health care consumerism. The investment in wellness programs is expected to provide a return on investment by a reduced number of accidents, decreasing expenses, and a decrease in the duration of disabilities and illness, thereby increasing the quality of life through improved health habits.

The cornerstone of the Health Services wellness strategy is the Health Assessment Program (HAP) which combines health risk appraisal, physical examination, laboratory analysis, and behavioral counseling. Nurses skilled in physical assessment and health behavioral modification see employees at two HAP sessions. Employees at high risk are further counseled, referred to intervention programs, and are given a follow-up date to return in order to chart their progress.

Active employees are eligible to repeat the program periodically based on age. HAP is offered at company medical facilities throughout the state, and for employees at distant locations, arrangements are made to "suitcase" the program. Accommodations are also made for employees with non-standard working hours.

The HAP database currently includes over 25 percent of all 62,500 active employees. Separate data systems contain information on sickness absence, about 10,000 cases annually; work injuries, about 2,500 cases annually; and medical costs for about 40 percent of all employees.

The four systems are integrated into a Health Intelligence Report System (HIRS). Data is presented showing how HIRS creates health profiles of Pacific Bell's business segments and measures the effects of health promotion on medical absence and health care costs.

Program results show reductions in major health risk factors and correlations between lower health care costs, program participation, and reduction of health risk.

In addition to this major program activity, employee health and fitness are fostered through a number of wellness programs whose range and scope are increasing. Automated machines for self-monitoring blood pressure are located throughout the company, and utilization is encouraged by periodic articles about high blood pressure and heart disease in employee publications. Weight scales are located with each blood pressure machine.

Mass cholesterol screenings are offered periodically using automated "fingerstick" analyzers. Participation is enhanced by educational material and by informational articles in employee publications.

The nutrition education program, "Food for Life," operates throughout all the company cafeterias, supported by employee publications. This has been made possible through a collaborative effort with the dining services staff and outside vendors. "Culinary Hearts"-style cooking classes are being planned.

The Health Information Program (HIP) was trialed in 1987 and will be expanded. The program offers non-prescriptive health information advice to employees, retirees, and dependents who are covered by the company's self-insured benefit plan. This service is provided to the employee by telephoning an 800 number that is staffed by a qualified Pacific Bell registered nurse.

The Employee Counseling Program (ECP), with a staff of nine licensed counselors, evaluates employees on a short-term basis about problems related to work, family, alcohol, drug abuse, and AIDS. Referrals to community resources are made when appropriate. A lunchtime seminar series on health-related topics is sponsored by the ECP.

Acquired Immunodeficiency Syndrome (AIDS) education is available to individual employees and work groups throughout the company by the ECP staff and other health professionals. Pacific Telesis Foundation was instrumental in the production of a video concerning AIDS in the workplace. The video, entitled "An Epidemic of Fear," is now used throughout the state. Education of employees concerning AIDS and substance abuse is a collaborative effort by union and management.

Stress management programs are offered through the Corporate Training Department and by the Health Services staff. A company psychologist provides Stress Awareness Training Seminars to employee groups on request or when a need is identified by supervisors.

Discounted memberships for fitness and weight control programs are available to active employees, and in some cases retirees and dependents, statewide. Employees who smoke may receive a discounted self-help program by calling an 800 number, and are also encouraged to use the programs of the American Lung Association and American Cancer Society. Outside vendors, such as Weight Watchers and Jackie Sorenson's Aerobic Dance, offer programs at the worksite on request.

In addition to the programs offered by Health Services, there are other wellness programs available to employees. For example, the Corporate Safety Department offers accident prevention and back health programs. Also, groups of employees throughout the company initiate wellness activities tailored to the particular needs and capacities of their work group. These include health fairs, running teams, aerobic dance competitions, newsletters, and invited speakers. The Health Service staff serve as consultants on these programs.

All of these wellness activities support the corporate commitment of valuing the individual and represent a business partnership to motivate optimum health in the workforce to meet the goals of the business. Information about the programs and their results are shared with the company officers on a regular basis and with other corporations through presentations at professional meetings and conferences.

PEPSICO, INC.

PepsiCo management believes "you can't run a successful company with half well people." The PepsiCo Health Enhancement Program implements that philosophy by motivating all employees and providing them with every opportunity to be healthy and fit.

PepsiCo is a major food and beverage service company. The divisions that most people know include Pepsi-Cola, Frito-Lay, Kentucky Fried Chicken, Pizza Hut, and Taco Bell. We also have about six other divisions which are not generally known here in the USA. They include Wine and Spirits and our International Foods and Beverages Divisions. In 1989, PepsiCo, Inc. grossed 13 billion dollars and employed approximately 235,000 people worldwide.

Reprinted courtesy of PepsiCo, Inc.

The major division headquarters offices consist of PepsiCo, Inc. at Purchase, NY, with approximately 700 people. The Pepsi-Cola division is in Somers, NY, and has approximately 1,200 employees. The Frito-Lay headquarters in Plano, Texas, has two major locations with 1,350 and 700 employees, respectively. Pizza Hut is in Wichita, Kansas, having about 800 employees on site, Taco Bell is in Irvine, California, with about 800 people, and Kentucky Fried Chicken is in Lexington, Kentucky, with approximately 800 people. All of the other locations for the company are described as field operations.

Each of the headquarters sites with the exception of Kentucky Fried Chicken, which we just recently acquired, have full service Fitness Centers and related Health Promotion Programs. The programs at each of the divisions are similar, but since we are a diversified company, there are individual variations based on interest, need and style of management.

Since the programs and facilities are similar, we will outline only one headquarter program as an example of what is done in each division.

At PepsiCo, Inc. headquarters in Purchase, NY, there is a 12,000-square-foot full service fitness facility. The equipment for this facility includes 12 treadmills, 16 bicycle ergometers (five arm/leg), four StairMasters, four rowers, one Gravitron, one recumbent cycle, 29 Nautilus stations, two complete sets of free weights, a twelve-station, variable resistance Universal machine, a separate 1,000-square-foot dance room with spring-loaded aerobic dance floor, and a full service in-house laundry.

In addition to this facility, space is leased at a nearby club and university for both indoor and outdoor swimming pools, indoor and outdoor tennis, racquetball, squash, and paddle ball which are all provided free to employees. Other recreation facilities and/or programs (i.e. golf) are made available to employees at service cost or at a discount.

Locker rooms provide the usual amenities which include whirlpools, saunas, and all toiletries. All employees are provided with towels, and an individual locker. They need provide only their shoes, since they can earn exercise clothing free, through the incentive attendance program. In addition, PepsiCo, Inc. has outdoor facilities which include jogging and walking trails, and bicycle riding areas. We have 12 outdoor bicycles for employee use. We also maintain a full stock of squash, tennis, and racquetball rackets for loan. There is an outdoor quarter mile track, softball field, volleyball court, and outdoor swimming pool and tennis court which are also available on our grounds. The organization recreation program includes basketball, volleyball, softball, ski club, runner's club, walking groups, bowling league, and soccer club.

All of these services are offered free to employees. Special programs of group exercise including aerobic dance and similar types of group activity have a minimal fee of $3 per session. The charge is designed to assure that people who sign up for the program will attend it. We offer a minimum of seven different classes at any one time with two in the morning, two to four at the lunch hour, two to four after work. The scheduling depends on demand and season of the year.

The Health Education/Lifestyle program is an extensive series incorporating all of the basic lifestyle format and related components as would be included in any Wellness Program. We have created a complete wellness environment. The cafeteria has a "lite," or low calorie food selection. Employees have flex times so they can exercise or attend Health education classes or participate in other special classes or health promotion activities (i.e. Health Fairs). Specifically, we offer courses and activities in the area of Behavior Change, Emotional Health and Medical Health. The behavioral change area includes: Substance Abuse, Nutrition and Weight Management, Stress Management, and Safety Education. Under Emotional Health, we include: Personal Development, Relating to others, Marriage, Divorce, Family and Children, Aging, and the Aged. Under Medical Health we include: Rehabilitation, Prenatal, Prevention and Screening, Disease Education, Emergency care and Medical services.

One of the most effective things is the integrated approach to the program which incorporates all levels of Wellness with a multi-year layout of what is to be offered. In addition, a coordinated effort is made to identify employee needs by working with Benefits, Medical, Personnel, and the Fitness Department.

This PepsiCo Health Enhancement Program is similar to the programs offered by our other major divisions of Pepsi-Cola, Frito-Lay, Taco Bell, and Pizza Hut. Each of our division headquarters houses one or more fitness centers with related health education programs.

In addition, we are undertaking Health Promotion programs with our field locations (i.e. plant employees, drivers, etc.). For example, our Frito-Lay Field Operations have four area Health Counselors who are responsible to help facilitate the development program in our 37 plants. We are developing fitness programs that hopefully will help reduce strain and sprain in our drivers. We are also investigating how health information can be effectively communicated to large groups of employee populations.

PepsiCo, Inc. has received numerous awards and recognition as a model program. Our purpose is to stay on the cutting edge of our fast-paced competitive business by providing programs that keep our employees healthy, fit, and productive.

PFIZER

Pfizer is a worldwide research-based company with businesses in healthcare, agriculture, specialty chemicals, materials science, and consumer products. The company employs approximately 40,000 men and women in an International network of 160 operating facilities in 60 countries. Pfizer World Headquarters is located in its Manhattan offices, home to over 3,000 employees.

Pfizer's Employee Health and Fitness Program was initiated at its World Headquarters in January 1986 under Pfizer's "Partners in Healthcare" theme. Partners in Healthcare is an appropriate summation of the program's philosophical approach requiring the cooperation of both staff and participant to accomplish the goal of improved health and well-being.

The Health and Fitness Center is a beautifully designed, state-of-the-art facility with a large exercise floor, group aerobics area, locker rooms, testing and therapy rooms, offices and conference rooms. It supplies a variety of services and programs, some of which are:

Reprinted courtesy of Pfizer.

- Comprehensive Physical Assessment
- Professional Staff Instruction and Supervision
- Personalized Exercise Prescription
- Aerobic Dance and Exercise Classes
- Cardiac and Orthopedic Rehabilitation
- Cardiovascular and Musculoskeletal Exercise Equipment
- Nutritional Counseling
- Weight Control Classes
- Stress Management Programs
- Smoking Cessation Programs
- Health Screening and Detection Programs

The facility is appointed with an impressive array of training, testing and therapy equipment.

Cardiovascular Exercise Equipment:

- Marquette Treadmills
- Universal Aerobicycles
- Universal Computerowers
- Monark Bicycle Ergometers
- Cybex Upper Body Ergometers
- Nordic-Trac Cross Country Ski Simulators

Musculoskeletal Exercise Equipment:

- Nautilus Weight Machines
- Cybex Eagle Weight Machines
- Universal Cable Weight Machines
- Universal Free Weights and Benches

Testing and Therapy Equipment:

- Q300 Stress Testing Monitor and Treadmill
- Physio-Control and 8 Channel Telemetry Monitor
- RJL Electrical Impedance Body Fat Analyzer
- Cybex 340 Extremity Training and Rehabilitation System
- Cybex 320 Electronic Digital Inclinometer
- Mens-O-Matic Minimal Electronic Non-Invasive Stimulator

- Bircher Megason 150 Ultrasound Unit
- Agar Transcutaneous Electrical Nerve Stimulator
- Transcutaneous Electrical Nerve Stimulator
- Hydrocollator Heat and Cold Pack Units

The Health and Fitness Center has a locker capacity for 600 members necessitating an age-down invitation system for enrolling members. The age-down system was preferred because of a greater correlation to an employee's years of company service and to development of cardiovascular risk factors.

The Health and Fitness Center offers both "Full" memberships and "Off-Peak" memberships. Full members have access to the facility from 6:00 A.M.–8:00 P.M., while Off-Peak members are limited to those hours in which the Center sees moderate utilization. There is a nominal fee assessed for each membership with the Off-Peak members paying approximately half of the Full membership fee.

The Health and Fitness Center offers Aerobic classes to the entire New York Office employee population. Creative scheduling and quantity of classes allows for an additional 1,000 employees to use the Center annually.

The Medical screening procedure prior to participating in the Health and Fitness Program is perhaps one of the program's most important assets. Medical history, cardiovascular risk factor profile, blood and urine analysis, resting electrocardiogram, pulmonary and respiratory function tests, and complete physical examination are completed by Pfizer's physicians (Board Certified Cardiologist). The Health and Fitness Staff then conducts an exercise stress test, nutritional assessment, percent body fat analysis, and a musculoskeletal assessment.

This information is used to design an individualized exercise prescription, indicate risk factors, and detect unknown health problems. For the latter, the testing procedures have been invaluable in uncovering cardiovascular disease in a number of individuals who required further medical testing and/or procedures. After completing the comprehensive physical, the member has an individualized program orientation. This orientation reviews all tests results, previews program involvement and discusses risk factor management. From this point the member proceeds into one of several recommended program tracks.

Asymptomatic healthy individuals with low to moderate risk factors enter the regular program. Individuals with moderate to severe risk factors, hypertension, cardiovascular disease or orthopedic problems are entered into a program or a combination of programs, to provide greater supervision and direction, with more frequent re-testing. Members who scored poorly on their nutritional assessments, are overweight, have poor blood lipid profiles or have health conditions that are in part managed by diet (diabetes, gout, cardiovascular disease, etc.) are assigned to the Nutritional Management Program.

Individuals with documented cardiovascular disease, history of cardiovascular complications or excessive risk factor profiles are entered into the Cardiac Rehabilitation Program. These members are monitored by telemetry while exercising and receive additional counseling on risk factor reduction. Stress testing and/or other tests relative to their condition will be performed every one to three months as indicated. Members with chronic or acute orthopedic problems are referred to the Orthopedic Rehabilitation Program. These members receive frequent testing and individualized training and if indicated may undergo treatment with one or more of the therapeutic modalities.

Hypertensive members are assigned to the Hypertension Intervention group. These members have their blood pressures checked daily and receive further consultation concerning medication, diet, weight reduction, and stress management.

In addition, the Health and Fitness Center sponsors health seminars and clinics in Weight Reduction, Smoking Cessation, Stress Reduction, Breast and Skin Cancer screenings, hypertension screen, etc.

The combined academic training and practical experience of the four Health and Fitness Center's staff members encompasses a wide range of health/fitness-related specialties including exercise physiology, cardiac rehabilitation, athletic training, orthopedic rehabilitation, nutrition, health education, physical education and program management. Their credentials are complemented by the expertise of two Board Certified Cardiologists and three occupational nurses on staff in the Employee Health Services Department.

Pfizer's Health and Fitness Center offers amenities such as hygienic supplies, exercise clothing, on-site laundry services, locker rooms and shower areas. It is an aesthetically pleasing and well-designed facility and it always is one of the stops on tours of the New York Offices given to visiting dignitaries, business associates, friends or family.

The success of the Pfizer Health and Fitness Program ultimately lies with its ability to supply valuable and convenient services through a variety of programs and thorough testing, managed by a professional staff and the support of Pfizer's management.

PROCTER & GAMBLE CO.

The Procter & Gamble Company manufactures and markets a wide range of laundry and cleaning products, personal care products, including pharmaceutical, food and beverage products, and a variety of products for business and industry. Procter & Gamble employs over 70,000 people worldwide.

Begun in July, 1985, Procter & Gamble's health promotion program, Lifestyle Decisions, provides employees and their families with the knowledge and resources necessary to understand the relationship between their lifestyles and health, and helps them make the changes that will lead to the happiest, healthiest state of well-being. Currently approximately 40,000 employees at 52 locations across the United States participate in the program.

The first phase of Lifestyle Decisions consisted of eight general education modules designed to increase employees' awareness of all aspects of a healthy lifestyle. Topics have included stress

Reprinted courtesy of Procter & Gamble Co.

management, auto and home safety, fitness and exercise, personal health care, nutrition, and cardiovascular health. The education sessions were supplemented by take-home materials (books, pamphlets, etc.) which provided additional information on the various topics.

Most materials for the program are developed in-house which allows for customization of the program to meet the particular needs of P&G employees. The program is administered by a core team at corporate headquarters. This team consists of two full-time staff members and one part-time physician. Outside consultants are also used as needed. The program is administered at the individual sites by a site facilitator, usually the site nurse.

As a result of the first phase of the program, various locations have begun on-site intervention programs in such areas as stress management, smoking cessation, and weight management. Several facilities conduct on-site aerobics classes, and a Corporate "Lifestyle Center" was opened at Corporate Headquarters in Cincinnati in September, 1987.

All of the Lifestyle education sessions are conducted on-site during regular working hours, at no cost to employees. Many of the intervention programs are also conducted on-site during company time, most with only a minimal charge to participants.

Phase II (begun January, 1988) focuses on creating a high level of awareness in two key areas—cardiovascular health and stress management. Employees and spouses are given the opportunity to complete a comprehensive Health Risk Appraisal that provides them with a confidential, personal report indicating individual risk factors and suggestions for improvement. In conjunction with the 1990 Health Objectives for the Nation as outlined by the U.S. Department of Health and Human Services, employees and spouses receive a cholesterol screening. Both the appraisal and cholesterol screen are free of charge to employees and their spouses.

From the data gathered from these reports, individual facilities receive aggregate data for their site showing the major risk factors for their employee population. From this aggregate data, intervention programs are established focusing on these risk factors.

TENNECO

Tenneco is a diversified company, headquartered in Houston, Texas with major interests in energy and manufacturing, employing over 90,000 employees worldwide. Principle businesses include: **Tenneco Gas Pipeline Group**—Operates a 20,000-mile network serving customers and 26 states from Texas to New England; **Newport News Shipbuilding and Dry Dock Company**—Of Newport News, Virginia is the largest privately owned shipyard in the world. Its main customer is the U.S. Navy for which it builds submarines and aircraft carriers; **Tenneco Automotive**—Is a worldwide automotive parts manufacturer and headquartered in Lincolnshire, Illinois comprised of three units: Walker exhaust systems, a retail division that includes Speedy Muffler King, Car-X and Pit Stop and Monroe shock absorbers; **Packaging Corporation of America (PCA)**—Headquartered in Evanston, Illinois is one of the largest producers of paperboard, molded fiber, aluminum foil, and plastic packaging with more than 50 plants in the U.S. and overseas. PCA also manages more than 450,000 areas of forest and is a leader of reforestation technology; **CASE-IH**—Formed in 1985 by a union of J. I. Case and International Harvester companies is headquartered in Racine, Wisconsin. CASE-IH is the second largest farm equipment manufacturer in the U.S. and is a leading manufacturer of small to medium size construction equipment; **Albright & Wilson**—Is headquartered in London, England and a major manufacturer of speciality chemicals.

The overall corporate culture of Tenneco is one of paternalism. Employment is generally stable with low turnover and generous benefits. This philosophy extends into the area of Health & Fitness.

The medical department was formed in 1981 by a desire of its chief executive officer to provide wellness programming for its employees. The program was developed as an employee benefit. However, the secondary goals were to attract applicants, assist in improving employee health and reduce absenteeism. Over the years, the company has funded much research to study the effects of wellness programs on productivity, health care costs, turnover, and absenteeism. The Health & Fitness program has become one of the trademarks of the corporation. The company is perceived throughout the world as one concerned about the physical condition and health of its employees.

HEALTH SERVICES

The Health Services Department is an on-site clinic for employees established in 1981 to provide preventive health counseling and education, surveillance, physical examinations and treatment of acute episodic illnesses with referral to community providers for chronic illnesses. The clinic is staffed by master's prepared advanced nurse practitioners who provide the primary care with consultation from staff physicians. The goal of the program is to promote wellness with emphasis on early intervention and treatment.

The health promotion program begins at the Health Services Department where a multiphasic screening program is provided to employees that includes biochemical laboratory analysis, spirometry, health history, physical assessment and a stress electrocardiogram for individuals over forty years of age. Each employee receives a health risk appraisal analysis which is discussed in a counseling session. During those sessions, current positive lifestyle behaviors are indicated and recommendations to improve health are made. A program is suggested for each participant through regular exercise and a well balanced diet with smoking cessation, stress management and drug and alcohol counseling when indicated. The goal setting process is then initiated with the identification of health habits that the employee is willing to begin to work toward changing. This process is reinforced following evaluation by the Health and Fitness Center staff.

The Wellness Program goal is to increase the employees' awareness and encourage them to take responsibility for their health and includes individual counseling, health screening and group education classes. All sessions are provided by the Tenneco staff and are scheduled during lunch or after hours at the Employee Center and at no charge to the employee. In the area of screening, hypertension, cholesterol, and glaucoma programs are provided annually. The cancer program consists of skin, breast, mammography, testicular and colorectal screening. Self-help programs include Overeaters Anonymous and Alcoholics Anonymous groups; weight reduction and smoking cessation contests; and a weight reduction program, "Eating Right," that includes a brochure for home use.

Group classes consist of smoking cessation, weight reduction, stress management, hearing conservation, nondrug treatment of hypertension, prenatal health, self-care, and cardiopulmonary resuscitation. In addition to these classes, a monthly seminar is presented that addresses current health issues. The Health Services Department provides primary care services to 85% of the Houston population each year. This helps the department stay in touch with the employee health needs and maximizes the health promotion opportunities.

HEALTH & FITNESS

The Tenneco Health and Fitness program was initiated in 1982 following the CEO's positive experience with exercise following bypass surgery. His major goal in establishing the program was to provide employees an opportunity to learn about and maintain positive health habits. An on-site health and fitness center was established which provides employees a convenient fully staffed exercise environment.

The Health and Fitness Center is located in an employee center, which also houses the employee cafeteria, a conference/training center, and executive dining room. Because of the many different activities which are offered in the employee center, it is an excellent location for the Health and Fitness Center. The center is 25,000 square feet, and is divided into five functional areas. There are locker rooms with dressing and wet areas. The wet areas have showers, saunas, and whirlpools. Four multi-use courts provide an area for racquetball, handball, and wallyball. The main exercise area contains over 30 pieces of Nautilus weight lifting machines, and an assortment of dumbbells. It also provides an open area for stretching, and the perimeter of this area is surrounded by 15 stationary bikes. A multipurpose room serves as the main exercise class room, and is also used for three-man basketball and volleyball. The largest and most used area within the health and fitness center is the 2/10 of a mile indoor track. The track is the largest indoor track in Houston and is 16 feet wide with each of the four corners banked slightly to relieve the tension of the turns.

In 1987, program membership was 2,169 employees, which represent 67% of the total downtown population (3,234). The average age of Tenneco employees in Houston is 32, and 75% of the program membership is less than 40 years of age. Males represent 60% of the total workforce and females 40%, whereas males are 53% of total health and fitness members and females 47%. The membership statistics are carefully monitored each month on a mainframe computer system. Upon entry into the center employees check in to the system which helps staff identify members and nonmembers. Following exercise participation employees log their exercise via terminals in the exercise area which provide immediate caloric expenditure feedback. This immediate feedback not only provides employees a way to quantify their exercise activities, but more importantly provides them instant motivation. Each month over 85% of the employees who exercise will log their exercise data, and 20% of this data is for exercise activity outside of the fitness center. A Monthly Activity Report is sent to all employees who have logged exercise and compares prior month exercise to current month, to year-to-date totals. It also helps employees track their body weight by providing beginning of the month and final monthly body weight.

The computer system has become an important management tool for program design, development, implementation, and evaluation. It allows staff to evaluate utilization of the different exercise activities, and the effectiveness of specific incentive motivation programs. The system also serves as a powerful marketing tool and can sort the membership population into many different interest groups and provide list and labels of these participants. Target marketing increases the effectiveness of the programming efforts, and allows staff to personalize their efforts.

Figure 1 illustrates program utilization, which counts the

FIGURE 1
1984–1987 Health & Fitness Center Utilization & Penetration

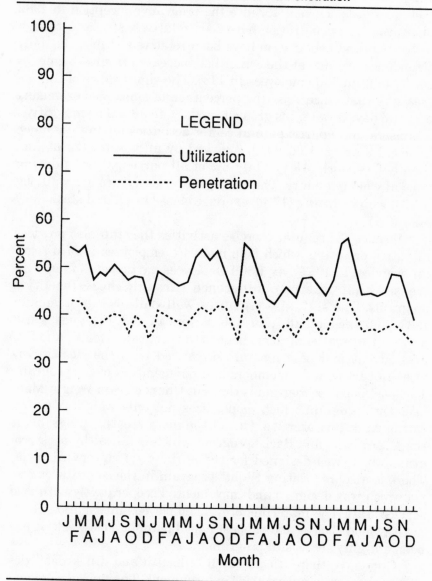

number of employees who exercise inside and outside of the center, and program penetration, which counts only those employees who exercise inside the center. Since the program's inception in 1982 utilization and penetration have been relatively stable. Although utilization and penetration have been relatively stable, the daily attendance average at the center has increased from 465 employees in 1982 to 530 employees in 1987. The significance of this increase is that since 1983 the percentage of employees exercising over two days a week has grown from 23% to 38%. The majority of exercisers (51%) participate in center activities during the lunch hour (11:00 A.M.–1:00 P.M.), followed by after work (23%), and then before work (18%). Only 8% of all participation is during normal working hours. The most popular activities are walk/jog (51%), weight lifting (17%), exercise class (14%), and stationary bike (6%).

Besides the regular exercise activities the staff also provides incentive programs which help motivate employees toward regular exercise. In 1987 over 1,500 employees participated in and increased their exercise adherence through these incentive programs. The staff also organizes wallyball (over 50 teams in 1987) and racquetball (over 150 players in 1987) leagues which provide a recreational component to the program. Health and Fitness educational programs are organized with the Health Services Department for members and nonmembers of the program. The most popular program is the "Fat Chance Team Weight Management" program which emphasizes not only weight loss, but eating right and exercise. One of the more creative programs is the "Hard Hats and Back" program which is a healthy back program which was designed for the offshore oil rig environment. There is also an "Eating Right" program in the company cafeteria which was designed and implemented cooperatively with food service staff. The materials provide employees information about healthy food choices and suggest a food plan for each week. It has been a highly successful program.

Currently, there are 15 satellite health and fitness facilities within the Tenneco worldwide environment. The information and ideas which are gained at the Houston program are shared and have been used effectively at these other locations. The health and fitness department strives to support and motivate Tenneco employees toward maintenance of healthier lifestyles with exercise as a major hook in the behavior change process.

THE TRAVELERS

Our new 48,000-square-foot facility houses a comprehensive lifestyle management program for Travelers employees, their families and retirees.

Through the Travelers' Employee Benefits Department and the Center for Corporate Health Promotion, the Taking Care Program has been designed to assist employees in making more informed decisions about their health, lifestyle and medical self-care. This is accomplished through an integrated and multi-faceted education and communications program—one that supports continuing employee participation within a framework of strong corporate support.

The Taking Care Center provides one-stop shopping in the area of prevention. The goals of the Travelers' Taking Care Center are to:

1. Enhance the health and decrease medical care costs of Travelers employees.
2. Improve productivity and morale of Travelers employees.
3. Provide visible evidence of the Travelers as a healthy, vigorous organization within the corporate community.

The Travelers' Taking Care Center is one of the largest corporate health promotion facilities in the United States. Included are a 25-yard indoor lap pool, sauna and whirlpool, walk/jog track, a wide variety of aerobic and strength training equipment, and a 3,000-square-foot dance room.

The ambience of the facility is very welcoming, offering warm colors, plants, and a contemporary interior design. Ease and convenience are of the utmost importance, with exercise clothing and daily laundry service provided for all participants. The membership fee of $12.00 per month is payroll-deducted over the course of the year.

A unique offering of the Taking Care Program is a strong health education component. In addition to a variety of exercise and activity classes, programs are offered in stress management, weight control, smoking cessation, nutrition education, prenatal classes, parenting, self-defense and healthy cooking.

Currently over 3,000 employees are actively using the Taking Care Center. All participants are involved in an initial screening process which includes assessments for blood lipids, aerobic capacity, body composition, strength, flexibility, and posture evaluation. From this information, individualized and goal-oriented exercise programs are designed for each member. Each participant's progress is monitored and strong motivation is provided for all members by the Taking Care Center's full-time professional staff.

A solid research effort has been developed to evaluate the effectiveness of the Taking Care Program. The research will examine the associations among health and health related characteristics and their effects on employee costs.

The Taking Care Program is offered to 38,000 employees throughout the country by the Center for Corporate Health Promotion and is distributed through the Taking Care newsletter, videos, brochures, tent cards and payroll stuffers. This cohesive and coordinated communications package delivers mutually reinforcing messages that foster healthy living.

UNISYS

Unisys offers its U.S. employees a number of health promotion opportunities programs, administered by physicians, nurses, exercise physiologists, psychological counselors, industrial hygienists, safety engineers and recreation specialists scattered throughout the country. Most of the Company's wellness programs are local

Reprinted courtesy of Unisys.

programs, financed and staffed by an operating group within Unisys and available at sites where there's a sizeable concentration of employees. Generally, more significant programs exist within Unisys Defense Systems unit and the engineering and manufacturing organization. In the past few years, some of these programs have been expanded or adapted into nationwide programs.

Historically, Unisys has focused on fitness facilities, educational workshops and major health-related events (e.g., health fairs). In some sites, the Company now is piloting new programs to encourage employees to lead healthier lives.

Workstation Invervention. In one program now being piloted, a health professional moves from work area to work area within a building, offering to measure employees' blood pressure, blood sugar and blood cholesterol. Test results are followed by a discussion of how to improve lifestyle habits to improve an employee's health.

The program has led to a higher rate of detection of elevated risk factors among employees, as well as success in modifying undesirable lifestyle habits—smoking, overeating, chronic inactivity—of employees.

Monthly Health Themes. Many of Unisys health programs use a varying health theme each month to educate employees (e.g., how to control dietary fat, how to minimize cancer risks, how to keep back problems in check). These themes are promoted through a variety of employee programs and individual consultations with Unisys health professionals. In addition, a monthly newsletter dedicated to health issues is sent to major U.S. employee sites.

Fitness Centers. Several major Unisys sites in the United States have fitness facilities. Other Unisys sites may have inhouse exercise classes or outdoor recreational facilities and organized activities.

Health Screenings and Assessments. For those Unisys sites with fitness centers, a variety of health screening and

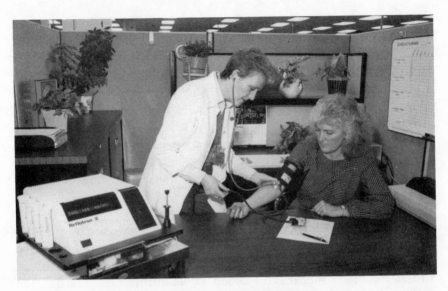

Employee participating in a regular blood pressure check at Unisys.

assessments may be available before the centers are used: a cardiovascular fitness test, body fat test, pulmonary function test. A computerized health risk analysis also is given to employees using the centers; results are interpreted by a qualified health professional. At some sites, a blood panel, muscular strength and flexibility analysis are included. Should a medical staff be available, employees also can obtain medical, optical and hearing screenings.

Health Promotion Workshops.   Some Unisys sites offer workshops and lectures on subjects such as weight management, nutritional habits, back care, stress and smoking.

The Future.   Unisys health professionals are continually seeking new solutions to providing opportunities for employee health enhancement. The program is therefore dynamic and constantly developing fresh approaches while maintaining time-honored protocols that work. Unisys looks forward to continued change and growth in this exciting field.

WARNER-LAMBERT

Warner-Lambert is a worldwide company engaged in the development, marketing and manufacture of quality health care and consumer products. The Company's diversified business portfolio encompasses ethical and non-prescription pharmaceuticals, chewing gums, breath mints and other confectionaries, shaving and pet care products and empty hard gelatin capsules. Corporate headquarters are located in Morris Plains, New Jersey. Approximately 7,000 employees are located in 10 locations throughout the United States and approximately 3,000 field sales employees.

MEDICAL SCREENING

While not a direct part of its health promotion program, Warner-Lambert's Medical Department provides free screening for blood pressure, cholesterol, cancer and glaucoma, etc. for all employees at the corporate headquarters. The Company uses its health promotion program to promote the screenings and encourage employees to maintain regular checkups for blood pressure and other types of conditions. At the plant site the Company uses industrial nurses to arrange for these screenings with the assistance of outside agencies.

The medical screenings are designed for early detection of disease or the potential for disease. For example, by providing its employees with the opportunity to participate in regular cancer exams, the Company hopes to detect a problem early and eliminate the employee anguish and stress if the need for major surgery arose due to an undetected malignancy.

At its headquarters, Warner-Lambert provides an Employee Assistance Program via a contractual agreement with a local hospital. Counseling, information, and referral are available to aid employees in a wide range of areas that might affect their personal lives such as family or marital difficulties, problems with alcohol or drugs, emotional problems, and financial or legal worries. This professional help is provided to Warner-Lambert employees and their families—confidentially and free of charge.

HEALTH PROMOTION

While early detection of disease is important, Warner-Lambert's health promotion activities emphasize prevention and employee wellness. Their health promotion program, entitled Life Wise, has five components: exercise, stress management, nutrition education, substance abuse and general health and self-care.

Corporate employees can participate in wellness seminars and special events. The seminars are conducted at lunch time by consultants in specialized areas of health promotion. Many of the presentations are conducted one hour a week for three to six weeks. The focus of the seminars has moved beyond the initial phase of awareness and concentrates on behavior change. Unique seminar topics include the following: "Take This Job And Shove It, " "Computing Your Nutritional Condition, " and "Living With Teens." Most seminars are free to employees or are offered at a nominal fee to encourage attendance in longer seminars.

In addition, one corporate-wide special event is conducted each spring and fall. A popular spring event has been a "Fun and Fitness Meet." In 1988, 19 teams of 12 employees each competed in fun activities such as a "Flipper Race," "Human Pyramid" and "Doubles Tennis With Racquetball Racquets." The meet was held on a Saturday at a nearby park with the assistance of a local YMCA. Points are awarded for the top finishers in each event with awards going to each participant on the top three teams.

A unique autumn activity is entitled the "Fall Fling." The event is a two-mile walk/run. Each registrant predicts the amount of time it will take him or her to cover the distance. All watches are removed prior to the start of the event. The top finishers are not necessarily the fastest runners, but rather those participants whose actual event time comes closest to his/her predicted time. Unique "Fall Fling" hooded sweat shirts are given to every finisher. In 1987, 230 employees participated in the after-work event organized by volunteers on Company outdoor parcourse.

Health promotion activities are conducted to various degrees at many of the domestic locations. Each location operates its activities with an independent budget but can utilize the Corporate Fitness and Health Promotion staff as a resource.

FITNESS CENTER

At its 13,500-square-foot Corporate Headquarters Fitness Center, Warner-Lambert provides locker and shower facilities, 62 stations of cardiovascular and weight-training equipment, a group exercise area and a 19-lap-per-mile indoor track.

Employees who want to participate in the fitness programs are required to go through a health screening. Depending on their risk factors they may be required to go through a complete cardiovascular stress test or a submaximal cardiovascular fitness assessment. Other components include a body fat percentage estimate and an assessment of low-back strength and flexibility. Based on a review of test results, the exercise test technician assists the participant in formulating fitness goals and develops a realistic individualized exercise plan. Then, each participant is provided with a complete orientation to the Fitness Center and its equipment.

Six full-time fitness professionals are on staff to regularly monitor each member's exercise progress. In addition, one college intern and five contract exercise instructors are available to monitor exercise sessions and offer suggestions, support and guidance.

Programming and incentives are an integral part of the success of the Warner-Lambert Fitness Center. Month-long events such as the "5 Lb. Challenge" and the "Cardiovascular Competition" have generated excitement and increased regular participation among the members. These activities along with a one-on-one personal touch are the characteristics identifying Warner-Lambert as a superior corporate fitness program.

Membership in the Fitness Center costs $10 per month. This includes health screening, along with center-provided towels, deodorant, shampoo, soap, etc. In addition, the center washes participants' workout clothing.

The Warner-Lambert program sells itself via quality programming and positive word of mouth. Currently, there are 950 members who average 240 visits per day. In addition, 350 additional employees are on a waiting list to become a member once capacity allows.

Although no fitness programs exist at any of the domestic locations, two sites are currently in the feasibility stage and many others do subsidize memberships at local exercise facilities. Most locations also sponsor recreational teams, such as softball and basketball, in local leagues.

The authors wish to thank Stephen Dover, Manager, Benefits Administration and Gene Babon, Manager, Health Promotion, for their assistance in the preparation of this report on Warner-Lambert's Health Promotion/Fitness Program.

WESTINGHOUSE ELECTRIC CORPORATION

Westinghouse Electric Corporation is a diversified, global, technology-based corporation whose goal is to increase the value of shareholders' investment through effective financial management, revenue growth, improved operating profit and effective asset utilization.

The principal business arenas of Westinghouse are television and radio broadcasting, defense and commercial electronics systems, financial services and the industrial, construction and electric utility markets.

Complementing these core businesses are operations serving selected "niche" markets such as vehicle transport refrigeration equipment, community development and beverage bottling.

Reprinted courtesy of Westinghouse Electric Corporation.

OUR PHILOSOPHY OF WELLNESS

Westinghouse's wellness programs reflect our diverse business activities. The corporation encourages each business unit within the company to adopt wellness programs that meet the needs, resources, and the demographics of that particular business and its employees. We provide a comprehensive training manual (*Sure Health Guide for Local Health Care Management*). In addition to workshops for wellness coordinators, a coordinator newsletter to share ideas, and coaching as needed, we also provide each location with an analysis of their health claims data so that they can see how much their location is spending on lifestyle-related illnesses. We believe that our decentralized approach, although slow to implement, builds on existing resources and efforts. Rather than being a corporate mandate, our efforts create a local ownership. This, we believe, is critical to the success of a strong, continuing program. The local approach also produces many creative possibilities for being about wellness—much more than could be generated with a single program.

Almost every wellness intervention exists someplace in Westinghouse, including eight in-house fitness facilities, health risk appraisals, cholesterol screening devices, newsletter, and comprehensive employee assistance programs. We even have had programs on snakebite prevention and earthquake preparedness!

THE SURE HEALTH LOCAL APPROACH TO FITNESS

Administratively, the *Sure Health* approach falls to two major categories, program management and specific health improvement action models. Program management involves the establishment of a local health care committee to oversee the health care needs of the particular work location and then select and implement those health care modules that are most appropriate. The specific health improvement action modules constitute a core of background information, guidelines, and references for use at the discretion of the local health care committee.

In addition to providing structure and visibility to health promotion programs, the local committee also serves as a vehicle for the dissemination of health care information to employees and dependents. Moreover, the local committee monitors health care utilization patterns to insure that the employees are using the most cost-effective medical services in the area when care is required.

Over and above these important functions, the local health care committee can also recommend ways to help implement corporate cost containment initiatives as well as encouraging appropriate use of local health care services.

The second component of the local health approach—the action modules—involves four principal categories:

- Risk Elimination
    Smoking cessation
    Alcohol abuse
    Drug abuse
    Hypertension control
    Stress reduction
    Immunization
- Fitness and Health
    Weight control
    Nutrition
    Exercise
    Jet lag
- Safety
    Seat belts
    Lifting
    Eye care
- Education
    Health lifestyle
    Prudent consumerism

On a regular basis, the Corporate Communications Department produces wellness articles and material for local newsletters. In addition, the Corporate Medical Director and the Headquarters Manager of Health Benefits can be contacted for additional source material for subjects that are not presently in the *Sure Health* manual.

One of the important features of the *Sure Health* approach is encouraging local committees to participate with local health care providers. For example, this involvement could include:

- Participation of the boards of directors of local hospitals or other health-related agencies.
- Membership on local health coalitions.
- Volunteering at local hospitals.
- Helping local hospitals set up quality circles or use Value Analysis.
- Lending expertise on energy management design or administrative procedures.

MANAGING RESULTS

Success of the *Sure Health* program at the local level ultimately depends on the leadership, endorsement, and support of local management. This support, however, is not always a given. In order to attract management's attention, committees are urged to report actual costs and key utilization factors to management on a monthly basis.

Some locations monitor success by comparing health care costs of exercisers versus non-exercisers. Other locations track the reduction of key risk factors (e.g., the percent of employees who smoke).

From a corporate viewpoint, wellness promotion is one of several actions to reduce health care costs. The other major actions address reducing unnecessary utilization, identifying preferred providers, and revising benefit plans to encourage appropriate employee use of health care services. Several factors are monitored at the corporate level to gauge progress. Three key factors which are monitored both corporately and locally are admission rates, hospital days, and cost-per-day. These macro-measures are easy to obtain and reflect the integrated results of all our actions. We recognize, however, that direct costs are only part of the benefit of wellness programs. There is more and more evidence that healthy workers lead to healthy companies, and our local committees often report considerable positive employee response to wellness.

THE WILLIAMS COMPANIES, INC.

The Williams Companies, Inc. is engaged in the pipeline transmission of natural gas and petroleum products, and interstate,
digital telecommunications.

The Company employs some 3,800 people, including approximately 1,400 in its headquarters offices in Tulsa, Oklahoma.

Williams' operating companies are:

- Northwest Pipeline Corporation, a 7,000-mile gas-
  gathering and interstate-transmission system serving
  seven western states.
- Williams Natural Gas Company, a 9,700-mile interstate gathering and transmission system serving six
  Midcontinent states.
- Williams Gas Marketing Group, a 470-mile pipeline
  system providing gas sales and transportation to the
  Louisiana industrial market. It is developing a nationwide presence as a natural-gas marketer.
- Williams Pipe Line Company, an 8,500-mile system
  providing transportation and distribution of petroleum
  products, liquified petroleum gas and crude oil in 10
  Midwestern states.
- Williams Telecommunications Group, one of the four
  largest fiber-optic telecommunications companies in
  the nation (in number of fiber miles). Williams Telecommunications provides nationwide private-line service to resellers and corporations.

THE WILLIAMS COMPANIES, INC. PHYSICAL
FITNESS/WELLNESS PROGRAMS PHILOSOPHY

The Williams Companies, Inc. can trace its ancestral roots directly to 1908. Imagine the puzzled looks on the faces of those
early-day bosses had someone asked them to describe their employee fitness/wellness programs.

Reprinted courtesy of The Williams Companies, Inc.

"Our what?" they probably would have replied.

The times have changed—for the good of both the Company and its employees. The mental and physical wellness of our employees figures heavily in the success we have achieved in operating our natural gas and petroleum pipelines, and in developing one of the nation's largest fiber-optic telecommunications networks.

"We believe that good-health programs for our employees actually save the Company money by providing greater productivity," says John Fischer, vice president of human resources. "We consider our many health programs as an investment, not a cost we can't recoup.

"Active, healthy people are sick less and present on the job more. They feel good about themselves, and they perform better," Fischer adds. "They react better to job demands, and they probably like their jobs better, too."

The Williams Companies provides numerous different health programs. A few examples:

- Diet programs where employees from one department may compete with employees from another area within the Company. Weekly weigh-ins are held at the nurse's station.
- Anti-smoking programs. One of our subsidiaries publishes the names of smokers who have quit for a certain number of months in its newsletter. Smoking is prohibited in many areas.
- Employee-conducted health risk appraisal, letting the employee know how he or she stacks up against the general population. For instance, a 45-year-old may learn that his health habits effectively place him at age 49. And vice-versa.
- Instructions on self-examination for breast cancer.
- Competitive sports, ranging from softball to bowling.
- Drug and alcohol-abuse programs.

The Company has introduced a program that provides off-site, confidential counseling for a wide range of problems—financial, marital, legal, etc.

"The counseling provides an employee with an assessment of any problem or challenge he or she may be facing," says Fischer.

"It also sends out a message—We care. We want to provide a channel for help because the sooner the employee receives help the sooner he or she can get back to a happy and productive life."

The Williams Companies' medical costs typically run below the national average. Company management from Chairman Joe Williams and President Vernon Jones on down gives some of the credit to the success of the ongoing health-care programs.

The Company health staff in Tulsa is comprised of Chris Bousum, manager of employee health/fitness; Myron Peace, manager of the health fitness center; Jill Hughes, fitness specialist; and Janice O'Brien, a registered nurse.

Bousum and Peace have master's degrees in physical education, while Hughes has a bachelor's degree in health education. All are members of the Association for Fitness in Business.

Bousum is certified by the American College of Sports Medicine as a preventive and rehabilitation-exercise specialist. Peace is a former Oklahoma state representative of the Association for Fitness in Business and has served on its four-state, regional board of directors. He served on the Oklahoma Governor's Task Force on Sports and Fitness for five years.

Together, Bousum, Peace, Hughes and O'Brien have 37 years of service to Williams employees.

Before the Company's corporate headquarters were moved into a new, 52-story building in downtown Tulsa in 1977, the concept of a health-fitness center already was taking shape. Interest grew, and the health fitness center opened in July 1978.

"It was the first corporate health fitness center in Tulsa and one of only a few in the region," recalls Peace.

Housed on parts of the 51st and 52nd floors, the center includes a 24-lap-per-mile track; a racquetball court and aerobic area in the center of the track; stationary bicycles, rowing machines and strength equipment; men's and women's locker rooms, each including whirlpool facilities; a food bar, where light-calorie breakfasts and lunches are served; and a fitness-evaluation room, where tests are performed involving cardiovascular capacity, body composition, strength, and range of motion.

All but one of the Company's five subsidiaries are located in Tulsa. Northwest Pipeline Corporation, headquartered in Salt Lake City, also has its own, on-site fitness center. The Salt Lake

City facility provides stationary bicycles, weight-training and rowing machines, a cross-country track trainer, and showers and locker rooms.

Senior Coordinator Marcia Gallenson and two part-time fitness specialists administer the Northwest Pipeline program. Gallenson, who holds a master's degree in health science, with an emphasis in exercise physiology, serves as the Utah representative for the AFB. She received the 1989 Outstanding Contribution to Fitness Award, which was issued by the Utah Governor's Council on Health and Physical Fitness.

Northwest Pipeline has received awards from the Utah Governor's Council on Health and Fitness four consecutive years, and has been named as a model for other work-site health programs in Utah.

At the fitness center, Northwest Pipeline employees earn personal awards as they continue regular exercise programs. They also take part in "Aerobicize Across the U.S.," where employees select and "travel to" a destination via aerobic-type exercises. They keep a record, charting their miles on a map in the facility.

Our Company's programs in Tulsa and Salt Lake City vary somewhat because of the different facilities, employee interests and logistics. However, the Company's fitness centers at Tulsa and Salt Lake City share the common bond of bringing employees together who otherwise might not get to know each other.

Larry Francisco, vice president of investor and public relations, says the centers repeatedly draw praise from employees because of convenience and the staffs' capabilities.

"If it's convenient, you can take the time during the work day to use it," Francisco says. "When I started going to our Tulsa fitness center 10 years ago, my back was in terrible shape. They helped me work that out. I think everyone realizes that healthy people do better."

Cindy Costa, supervisor of executive support for The Williams Companies, praises the center for the break it provides in her routine.

"It's wonderful just to get away from your desk," she says. "The center helps me feel that we all are on the same team. We make new friends, and we feel better—physically and psychologically."

Similar praise is heard at Salt Lake City. "Every company in America should have a program like this one, " says Sue Calegory, senior financial analyst for Northwest Pipeline, who reports that she has lost weight, improved her health, and lowered her stress level.

Chris Bousum says Company employees at all locations are being taught to "assume responsibility for their health, and turn negative health behaviors into positive health behaviors. We view the major diseases as, in effect, 'diseases of choice' because they can be prevented in many cases. One of our goals is to help employees make the right choices to avoid diseases, which affect them, their families, friends and the Company.

"The common denominator in all our programs—whether it's sponsoring a noon discussion on how to prevent job burnout or supporting the nationally popular 15-kilometer Tulsa Run each fall—is that we want to improve the quality of life for our employees, both personally and professionally," Bousum says. "It's a win-win situation."

W. R. GRACE & CO.

W. R. Grace & Co. is an international specialty chemicals company with selected interests in energy manufacturing and service businesses. Grace operates more than 1,300 facilities and employs approximately 45,700 people in 44 countries. Grace is headquartered in New York City where it employs 531 people.

FITNESS FACILITIES

The physical and mental well-being of every employee is a top priority at Grace. To encourage physical fitness, the Company provides headquarters employees with fully equipped, free-of-charge, exercise facilities. The gym is equipped with:

Reprinted courtesy of W. R. Grace & Co.

- Universal Weights
- Free Weights
- Stationary Bicycles
- Nautilus Abdominal Machine
- Computerized Treadmill

The gym, which is open from 7:00 A.M. to 7:00 P.M., Monday through Friday, is located on the fifth floor of the Grace building, making its use convenient to Grace employees.

Grace management fully supports employee involvement in exercise activities, believing that a corporate fitness program enables a company to provide the following:

- An increased feeling among personnel that the Company is concerned for their well-being. This feeling develops greater loyalty on the part of the employees.
- An increased level of health and fitness, decreasing absenteeism, serious illness, and job stress, and increasing productivity.

In addition to the exercise facilities, Grace also sponsors a softball league with approximately 100 employee participants, a running club and subsidies for aerobic classes.

Upper management support for health and fitness is reflected in the appearance of senior officers, generally very fit and trim.

MEDICAL DEPARTMENT

A fully staffed Medical Department is also available to employees for first aid treatment and routine laboratory examinations such as blood tests and X rays, as well as consultation on health matters concerning employees or members of their immediate families.

EMPLOYEE ASSISTANCE PROGRAM

To help employees with personal problems which can affect health, relationships and job performance, Grace provides a free Employee Assistance Program. Under this program, employees can

Office Bulletin No. 2566

March 2, 1989

Memorandum to All Employees

Physical Fitness

Membership in nearby health clubs is quite costly. Here at Grace, employees have the opportunity of using the company physical fitness center **FREE OF CHARGE.**

Today's media is replete with reports on the personal health benefits that emanate from regular physical exercise. Just thirty minutes of exercise several times a week can pay huge dividends in terms of one's general health.

Grace's 5th floor gymnasium has a wide selection of equipment designed to help all employees keep in shape. There is something for everyone, including:

— Universal gym
— Universal leg lift
— Universal arm lift
— Universal treadmill
— Universal Roman chair
— Monark cycles (2)
— Precor rowing machine
— Nautilus abdominal machine
— Barbells and weight bench
— Assorted dumbbells
— Jump rope

In addition, based upon the input we received from the employees who attended our open meeting last November, some *new equipment* has just been added:

— Bodyguard 990 Ergometer Mark II cycles (2)
— Lower weight dumbbells (10 and 5 lbs)
— Weight bench

If you would like the opportunity to familiarize yourself with the physical fitness facility and the equipment, come to the special **FAMILIARIZATION SESSION** that will be held in the gymnasium at 11:00 a.m. on Tuesday, March 7th. Some of the employees who utilize the equipment on a regular basis will be on hand to explain how each apparatus works and the physical benefits that result from its use. Gym clothes are not necessary for this session.

All employees are encouraged to "Get in shape!" Come and use the **FREE** physical fitness center any weekday between 7:00 a.m. and 7:00 p.m. Lockers and showers are available.

T. M. Lawlor

access completely confidential, professional assistance with personal problems 24 hours a day, seven days a week for short-term counseling or referral to a professional agency for assistance.

SECTION 3

THE MEDICAL ASPECTS OF FITNESS/WELLNESS PROGRAMS

William S. Frankl, M.D.

Central to the implementation and successful operation of a fitness/wellness program is an understanding of what constitutes "wellness" and what it means to be "fit." In this section William S. Frankl, M.D., discusses such important areas as the need for pre-exercise physical examinations, exercise precautions, warm-up, use of aerobic and nonaerobic exercises, and establishing individual exercise programs. He also addresses smoking, hypertension, weight control, cholesterol, alcohol, and diet. Every manager, as well as all of those employees who participate in fitness/wellness programs, should carefully study this section.

CONTENTS

Management Overview
Medical Introduction
Fitness, Aerobic, and Anaerobic Exercises—Warm-Up and Heart Function
Physical Examinations and Exercise Precautions
What Every Manager Needs to Know about Smoking, High Blood Pressure, Weight, Cholesterol, Alcohol, and Diet
Stress and "Type A" Behavior
Preparing Children for Good Health

MANAGEMENT OVERVIEW

> Truth often suffers more
> by the heat of its
> defenders than from the
> arguments of its
> opposers.
> *William Penn*

Popular literature provides extensive information about health, fitness, exercise, and diet. Unfortunately, our research indicates that much of this is confusing and sometimes inaccurate. In the following section, William Frankl, M.D., a renowned cardiologist, provides accurate and up-to-date information that every manager should have and utilize in his or her personal life and in encouraging employees to be healthy. Clearly presented facts go a long way in helping people modify their behavior.

In our research we also noted that some companies do not yet provide the kinds of extensive physical examinations recommended by Dr. Frankl. Thus, we recommend close consideration of his advice when implementing and conducting fitness/wellness programs.

MEDICAL INTRODUCTION

> Life is like riding a
> bicycle. You don't fall
> off unless you stop
> pedaling.
> *Claude Pepper*

This book describes the hundreds of corporate wellness/fitness programs that are provided by companies throughout the country. When operated by knowledgeable specialists, these programs can offer great opportunities for employees at all levels to manage their own health in an educated manner. *Education is the key to proper self-health management.* Let's see why.

If you look at medicine in America in the 18th and 19th centuries, doctors were generally held in low esteem because there really wasn't very much they could do for their patients. There was substantial interest in "natural" treatment of disease. For example, if you had tuberculosis, you were put in a sanitarium, where a clean, cool environment existed. Sanitariums were built at high elevations where the air was thought to be clean, the idea being that clean air would clean out the lungs. Obviously, that whole idea was totally incorrect.

Doctors used natural herbs and potions. That was probably appropriate because they did neither harm nor good. But they may have helped patients psychologically. Since there really wasn't much a doctor could do, and a lot of things doctors did were quite harmful, such as using leeches for treating typhus fever, people sought their own remedies or "cures."

In the 20th century, technology really took hold in the medical field. The engineers, biochemists, and physicians, and later with the advent of computers, all came together to produce enormous changes. The technological advances truly have been astonishing. Mozart might have survived to be 90 had he lived in the latter one third of this century. Beethoven might not have been deaf because he might have had a cochlear transplant.

But the medical community, with the help of the media,

oversold itself. The American public began to believe and insist that we could treat anything successfully. Unfortunately, that is just not the case. We can't successfully treat every disease. In fact, medicine is on a plateau right now. We are looking for the next big breakthrough in molecular biology which will take us into the 21st century.

In addition, we make mistakes. We are not 100 percent correct all of the time. Clearly, the medical field was oversold, and now the American public is becoming disenchanted.

Also, computers have come between doctors and their patients. The computer has tended to depersonalize the doctor-patient relationship. The reason is that doctors can often learn a great deal more about the patient's physiology from the analysis of a vial of blood than they can from talking with their patients, or at least many physicians believe this is so. However, a doctor can learn many important things during a conversation. Thus, our technology actually has produced a rift between doctors and patients.

The overselling of medicine, combined with the cooling of doctor-patient relationships, have led many people to adopt a "do-it-yourself attitude" toward medicine. We are witnessing a swing back toward a kind of self-treatment folk medicine—the "apple a day keeps the doctor away" approach. This folk medicine approach had led, for example, to the opening of thousands of health food stores and numerous publications on preventive and curative medicine based on limited and often inaccurate data.

This folksy approach to prevention and cure, based on misconceptions and myths, can be dangerous. Taking fish oil supplements, for example, with the hope of reducing one's cholesterol may actually be ineffective, and may be dangerous. Starting an exercise program without first having an appropriate physical examination may prove fatal. Exercise can kill you if you do it and you're not fit to do it.

What should people do, then? *People should take an active, educated approach to self-care.* Certainly, one can't be passive and just depend on a physician. But, the approach to improving individual health must be an educated one, not a folk-medicine approach. An educated population—educated by knowledgeable people—will enjoy better health.

The primary purpose of corporate fitness/wellness programs is to get people involved in their own health management, but in an informed manner. When operated by knowledgeable specialists, fitness/wellness programs can make an important contribution to the health of Americans.

FITNESS, AEROBIC, AND ANAEROBIC EXERCISES— WARM-UP AND HEART FUNCTION

> Look to your health; and if
> you have it, praise God, and
> value it next to a good
> conscience. For health is a
> blessing that money cannot
> buy.
> *Izaak Walton*

1. *From a medical viewpoint, what does it mean to be physically fit?*

Physically fit people, who are well-toned and developed, rather than flabby, generally have a leaner body mass and muscles that utilize oxygen more efficiently. This means a lesser load on the heart. Also, if you are physically fit, you can exercise at a lower heart rate and perform any physical activity more efficiently. From a medical standpoint, therefore, it certainly is better to be physically fit.

2. *Which types of exercises do you recommend and why? Are there any that you would not recommend?*

Exercise can be grouped in two categories: *aerobic and anaerobic.* Aerobic exercises include such activities as bicycling, dancing, swimming and walking at a brisk pace. Aerobic exercises produce an increased return of blood to the heart.

For example, in swimming or bicycling, you are pumping your legs. This results in an increased blood flow in the veins and into the right side of the heart, after which blood is then pumped out of the left side of the heart. *When you are doing aerobic exercises, you are providing the heart muscle with increasing amounts of blood, and that increases the cardiac output.*

With aerobic exercises, you raise your systolic pressure and decrease your diastolic pressure. During these exercises, the mean pressure in your aorta is about the same as when your body is at rest. The heart muscle is expanded with the increased volume of incoming blood. Then, with each contraction, the heart is able to put out an increased volume of blood in order to provide the appropriate flow of blood to exercising muscles, the brain, the heart, and so forth.

The other category of exercises—*anaerobic exercises*—most typically is found in weight lifting. When you lift weights, planting your feet on the ground and using your arms to lift the weights, you are not increasing the flow of blood back into the heart. Lifting weights, in fact, produces a big increase in the resistance in the aorta. As this resistance rises, the heart has to work harder, since it has to provide an increased supply of blood to the upper portion of the body.

With increased pressure in the aorta, the heart demands more oxygen so that it can deliver more blood forward as it pumps against increased resistance. This demand isn't met, however, because the heart is not getting an increased supply of blood by venous return from the lower portion of the body. *Anaerobic exercises require more oxygen and more cardiac output without providing more blood to the heart. In addition, these exercises increase the resistance of the heart muscle to ejection of blood.*

I advise engaging in aerobic exercises and avoiding those exercises which are clearly anaerobic (stationary kinds of exercise). In addition to weight lifting, other kinds of anaerobic exercises include pushups, situps, and pulling weights on pulleys. All of these are, more or less, oxygen using and do not provide the needed blood flow back through the cardiovascular system.

Anaerobic exercises certainly do build up muscles; however, you also can build muscle by swimming, which builds up both leg and arm muscles. Similarly, bicycling will do a great job with your leg muscles and, like swimming, is an aerobic exercise. For the general population, no better exercises can be prescribed than swimming, bicycling, hiking, or dancing. They are all very good.

Athletes, who need to develop special muscle groups, may want to do anaerobic exercises. But, these people should heed the cautions noted above and certainly go through a series of aerobic warm-up exercises first.

3. *When you were discussing good aerobic exercises, you did not mention jogging. What is your opinion of jogging?*

Although jogging is an aerobic exercise, I don't recommend jogging for several reasons. First, people generally do it alone. Furthermore, they often do it in isolated places or along roads. If they do have underlying heart disease, the possibility of sudden death exists. Jim Fixx is a tragic example. Often, no one is around to help a person jogging in an isolated area nor is there anyone who will stop to assist a jogger in distress along a road.

Second, jogging is bad on the spine and the knees. The spinal column is subjected to a great deal of trauma and the knees take punishment, too. So, I am not a great fan of jogging. But, if you were to ask me if it is better to jog than to weight lift, I would say it is clearly better to jog.

4. *Is there any difference between jogging and running?*

Running is more limited in that the pace is faster and a person tends to give out sooner.

5. *To maintain good cardiovascular condition, how frequently and for how long a period should a person exercise?*

This is a difficult question to answer and depends upon the person's physical condition, as well as any history of heart disease. For those with any form of cardiovascular disease, cardiac physiologists recommend exercising about three times a week for optimum improvement. But, the exercise is clearly heart-rate dependent.

If a person has had a heart attack and is now in a rehabilitation program, the initial exercise should be designed to achieve a target heart rate around 10 beats per minute higher than the *resting heart rate.* (A person's resting rate is the pulse rate taken with the person standing upright but not moving.) For those who have had bypass surgery, their target heart rate should also be about 10 beats per minute above the resting level.

After a patient has been training for some period, the level of oxygen he or she is using when exercising should be measured. This provides a baseline. Then, the physician targets an increase in oxygen consumption 60 to 80 percent above the baseline exercise rate. In those instances when it is not possible (or feasible) to measure oxygen utilization, the physician targets an increase in pulse rate of about 60 to 80 percent above the resting heart rate. In all cases, an individual assessment taking into account age as well as possible underlying heart disease must be considered when establishing a target heart rate.

For the normal individual (the person who has not had any incidence of heart disease), he or she should have a stress cardiogram before starting an exercise program. (Pre-exercise medical testing and evaluation are discussed below.) At that point, it is usually possible to determine if the individual has had any cardiac disease.

If the person's exercise test is perfectly normal and his or her tolerance for exercise is good, the physician will tell the person what level of exercise likely can be attained without the development of significant fatigue. The physician also will plan an exercise program based on the results of the exercise test. Establishing an exercise program is an individualized procedure.

With respect to frequency and duration of exercise, about three times a week for half an hour is a good target.

6. *Is there an optimum heart rate a person should attain?*

There is no optimum heart rate a person should attain. The target heart rate depends upon the individual's resting heart rate. Attaining an increase of 60 to 80 percent over the resting heart rate is a good target. But, as noted above, the target is a function of the results of the exercise test and varies from person to person.

7. *With respect to cardiovascular function, how important is "warming up" before exercising?*

Very important. Warming up distributes blood through the working muscles. If you don't warm up, you will fatigue much more rapidly, since you won't have allowed time to get the needed blood to your muscles. Also, in the warm-up period, you stretch some of the ligaments, which helps to reduce the risk of ligament injury. *Walking at a brisk pace for two or three minutes is a good warm-up.*

8. *What should a person's target heart rate be during aerobic type exercises? Does this vary with age?*

The target rate should be somewhere in the range recommended by the American Heart Association. It varies from person to person and, as noted earlier, depends on age and the possibility of underlying heart disease.

9. *If the person doesn't achieve the American Heart Association's target heart rate, is the person getting very much out of the exercise?*

Sure. I think there is a misconception that you have to reach some defined targets. We all differ very markedly in our exercise capacity, which varies with age and a number of other factors. *Clearly, a little exercise, whether a target heart rate is reached or not, is better than no exercise at all.*

PHYSICAL EXAMINATIONS AND EXERCISE PRECAUTIONS

> Health and cheerfulness mutually
> beget each other.
> *Joseph Addison*

1. *If a person has not been exercising regularly, how extensive a physical examination should the person have before starting an exercise program?*

This is an extremely important question, especially the older a person is. Let's consider first the person who is exercising regularly and is in good shape. The person, let's say, is 40 to 50 years old. He or she has been playing singles tennis for a long time, perhaps skis or swims, and is generally in good shape. This is the ideal person. To interfere with that person's program is unreasonable, although with advancing age, a person must become more cautious about the length and vigor of the exercise. One never knows if silent coronary artery disease may be present.

The individual who has not been exercising regularly should undergo an exercise cardiogram. This test will indicate if the blood pressure response to exercise is appropriate. The systolic blood pressure should rise while the diastolic pressure falls. But some very hypertensive people may show a precipitous rise in the systolic and diastolic pressure. This puts an enormous amount of stress on the heart.

Next, the physician examines the cardiogram during the exercise test and looks for any indications of abnormality in the blood flow through the coronary arteries, suggesting a lack of blood flow to the heart muscles. Such a lack of blood flow back to the heart muscles is clearly a reason to hold back on the person's exercise. The physician also determines how long the person can exercise, the point where fatigue sets in, and the heart rate at that point of fatigue. The person would be directed to stay below that heart rate when exercising.

To summarize, a person should start with a complete physical examination, including blood pressure measurement and a resting cardiogram. If the results are satisfactory, then the person should proceed to a stress cardiogram. If the stress test is abnormal, then a stress test and a thallium scan, which is more precise in terms of picking out coronary artery disease, is indicated. If the individual has a negative stress test or negative stress and thallium test, the person can go on to a prescribed exercise program appropriate for his or her age.

2. *Does everyone, such as a 20-year-old, need as extensive a physical examination as you described above?*

It depends on family history. If the person has a family history of heart attacks and/or strokes, he or she should go through the extensive exam described above. If the person does not have such a family history, then testing beyond a routine physical examination, including a chest X-ray, blood pressure testing, heart activity monitoring, including a resting cardiogram and some blood studies, including blood sugar and blood lipids, probably is not necessary. All of these routine tests provide clues to the possible existence of silent heart disease and should be obtained, even in young persons, without a significant history of cardiac disease.

3. *How can a person tell if he or she is exceeding safe limits of exercise participation?*

Some people can't. Possible signs of exceeding safe limits include excessive shortness of breath, constriction(s) in the chest and muscle aches (most frequently in the leg muscles). If a person experiences any of these, he or she should stop. If the person experiences excessive shortness of breath or chest constriction, he or she should see a doctor.

4. *What is "excessive shortness of breath"?*

This is very nebulous. If a person is very well-conditioned, breathing is much more relaxed and much less rapid than a poorly conditioned person. If a person is poorly conditioned, he or she is likely to become very short of breath very quickly. This increase in the rate of breathing is the body's way of trying to deliver oxygen more efficiently to the heart.

5. *After exercising, how fast should the heart rate decrease?*

If it takes longer than five minutes for the person's heart rate to return to normal, we usually think the person is in very poor physical condition, or they have occult (undetected or not very obvious) congestive heart failure.

6. *Are there particular times when exercise should be avoided (such as during warm or cold weather)? Should special precautions be taken in the cold?*

Yes. When the weather is cold, the blood vessels in the skin, as well as the vessels in the muscles, constrict to preserve heat. Any time the heart is put under any stress (such as when exercising), a protective mechanism comes into play that shunts blood to the brain, the heart muscle itself, and also to the kidneys. In very cold weather, the muscle and skin vessels contract. This raises the resistance in the aorta, forcing the heart to beat against increased pressure and consequently increasing the need for oxygen. So, if the individual has underlying heart disease, he or she is at much greater risk.

On the other hand, in very hot weather, all of these vessels dilate tremendously to get rid of heat. This causes vascular resistance to fall very markedly. When a person exercises in hot weather, an increase in the return of blood to the heart, coupled with reduced vascular resistance, forces the heart to work harder. So, for both very cold and very hot weather, the heart is put under much more stress.

I am very upset when I see a person jogging on a day when the wind is blowing and the temperature is 20 degrees. The same is true when it is 90 degrees, the sun is out, and the humidity is high. I have observed that when there are marked turns in the seasons, there seems to be an increased incidence of heart attacks and sudden death. These climatic conditions place a greater stress on the heart.

7. *How long after eating should a person wait before exercising?*

This depends to a large degree on the presence of any underlying heart disease. After eating, blood is shunted to the gastrointestinal tract to help with digestion. Because of that, I generally recommend an hour or two waiting period. By this time, digestion has been completed and the shunting has ceased.

8. *Can exercise offset the harmful effects of smoking?*

No!

WHAT EVERY MANAGER NEEDS TO KNOW ABOUT SMOKING, HIGH BLOOD PRESSURE, WEIGHT, CHOLESTEROL, ALCOHOL, AND DIET

> To wish to be well is part
> of becoming well.
> *Seneca:* Phaedra

1. *Considering the factors that can increase the risk of heart disease such as smoking, high blood pressure, being overweight, having high levels of cholesterol, alcohol consumption, etc., which do you consider to be the most important?*

Number one, without any question and far above any others, is smoking. It is rare to see a patient with significant coronary heart disease who has always been a nonsmoker. It happens, but certainly not very often. Experimental studies show that the tars and nicotine can directly injure blood vessels. *I also want to emphasize that passive smoking is almost as bad as actual smoking.* Sitting in a plane next to someone who is smoking, or sitting in a room with someone who is smoking, is almost as bad as smoking yourself. It is a tragedy that the tobacco industry is subsidized by the same federal government that pays billions of dollars in health care costs for patients with coronary heart disease and lung cancer.

Number two is high blood pressure. When a person has high blood pressure, the heart has to work harder. The muscle squeezes more vigorously. This extra-vigorous contraction may produce mechanical kinking of the coronary arteries as they go from the surface of the heart down into the heart muscle and produce damage at the "bend" in the vessel, thus allowing cholesterol to infiltrate into the walls.

The third is high levels of cholesterol. Smoking, high blood pressure, and elevated cholesterol are the "big three," along with diabetes. Patients who are diabetic tend to have accelerated coronary artery disease.

Being overweight in and of itself, as an isolated factor, is not a great risk factor for coronary artery disease. But, we must note that a person who is overweight is more likely to have an elevated cholesterol level, high blood pressure, and also to be a smoker. Generally, it is these other factors surrounding the overweight person that are the hallmarks of coronary heart disease. The famous longitudinal Framingham study indicates that being overweight, if none of the other risk factors are present, is not extremely important in and of itself.

Small doses of *alcohol*, perhaps two ounces of hard liquor or four ounces of wine taken daily, tend to raise the level of high density lipoprotein cholesterol (HDL)—which is good. Small doses of alcohol also tend to lower the level of low density lipoprotein cholesterol (LDL)—which is also good. Thus, there seems to be some evidence that small amounts of alcohol may be beneficial in reducing cholesterol. *However, alcohol clearly depresses the heart muscle (i.e. it causes the heart muscle to contract less vigorously and less normally) and may actually be injurious to the heart muscle.* Some forms of heart disease result from excessive ingestion of alcohol; therefore, I am not advocating alcohol. Alcohol can also damage the liver. Alcohol does not increase a person's risk of coronary disease. Rather, it is a risk factor in other forms of heart disease.

At this juncture it is important to make clear distinctions among the various types of heart disease. In the popular media, we see a lot about preventing heart disease. That is like saying, "preventing getting sick." All of the popular literature which speaks to preventing heart disease is really talking about coronary artery (or coronary heart) disease. Clearly, smoking, high blood pressure, high cholesterol, and diabetes are risk factors for coronary artery disease, as well as for vascular diseases and stroke. But they are not risk factors for valve disease or cardiomyopathies or congenital heart disease. *People who smoke, have high blood pressure and high cholesterol levels are at a greater risk for stroke and coronary heart disease.*

2. *If a person has high blood pressure and wants to reduce salt in his or her diet, what would you recommend?*

I give people some very simple guidelines. Throw out your salt shaker! Avoid pretzels, potato chips, salted nuts, and salty junk food. If you avoid these, you will be on a moderately low salt diet.

A couple of years ago a report from the Department of Health and Human Services suggested that everyone should be on a low salt diet. This cannot be translated to apply to an entire population. The fact is that if you have a family history of high blood pressure, or are currently suffering from high blood pressure, then you should be on a low salt diet. Otherwise, you don't need to avoid salt.

The fact is that eating is an important part of living. If you make the food tasteless, many people will not follow even a prudent diet. They will be so miserable they will decide that they would rather be dead or have a stroke rather than eat tasteless food.

I think you can be awfully miserable by doing what some health proponents put forth today. You feel guilty about eating some meat when at a party or using some butter at a restaurant, when, in fact, that is the only butter you used all week. Moderation, not guilt, is the answer to dieting.

3. *The medical community recently recommended that everyone maintain cholesterol levels below 200. Do you support this recommendation, or can the level vary with age?*

This is a very complicated question. It is all very well and good to say that an individual's cholesterol should be under 200. From the standpoint of the population as a whole, from a purely statistical viewpoint, that is, it is clear that the lower a person's cholesterol, the lower the likelihood of having a coronary event (an acute heart attack or sudden death). A level of cholesterol under 200 is therefore better than one over 200.

As far as age goes, I am astonished to see people who are in their 70s and 80s who have been told by their doctors that their cholesterol is, say, 250 and that they therefore should go on a low cholesterol diet. If you reach the age of 70 or 80, and you haven't had a major cardiac event, but your cholesterol is 300, so what!

These recommendations can be interpreted as generally applicable to the American population as a whole. They are simplistic, however, inasmuch as the cholesterol question has many other aspects, including the fact that *total cholesterol is not the significant factor in most cases*. Generally, we find that if a person has a level of cholesterol under 200, the level of high density lipoprotein cholesterol (HDL) is likely to be high—which is good. Also, the level of low density lipoprotein cholesterol (LDL) is likely to be low—which is also good. However, if a person has a cholesterol level *over 200* and also has a high level of HDL and a low level of LDL, he or she is unlikely to be at risk.

It is clear that the development of coronary heart disease is lower in those who have lower cholesterol. But this is again simplistic. If your cholesterol is 201, would you say that is bad? What about a level of 199? Is that good? Obviously, small differences are not important. When evaluating a person's cholesterol, other risk factors should also be taken into consideration. For example, if you are a nonsmoker and nondiabetic, someone who is lean and also exercises, with a good family history, a cholesterol level of 220, 230 or 240 is probably much less meaningful.

On the other hand, if your cholesterol is 170 or 190 and you are diabetic, overweight, a smoker, and you have a bad family history, your "low" cholesterol level may also be much less meaningful. In this example, a low cholesterol level isn't particularly important in your total cardiac health picture because you have all those other risk factors playing much more significant roles.

Many of the studies recommending the maintenance of a cholesterol level below 200 are population studies. The Japanese, for example, used to have a lower level of coronary artery disease than found among Americans. The Japanese also had low levels of cholesterol—in the 130 to 140 level. Certainly their diets resulted in these lower levels and by changing diet many people can reduce cholesterol levels.

The cholesterol level in the blood is a combination of what you produce yourself plus what you eat. In some cases, it may be impossible to reduce the amount of cholesterol by changing dietary patterns, even if you starve yourself, because the body will continue to produce high levels. In these instances, drugs for reducing cholesterol, such as the new Lovastatin (brand name, Mevacor) and an older drug called Cholestyramine Resin (brand name, Questran), may be prescribed.

What do I tell my patients? I tell them to try to be prudent about their diet. If they have a bad family history, if they high blood pressure, and certainly if they are diabetic and have any evidence of coronary artery disease, I try to emphasize the need to get their cholesterol down.

It is still unclear whether or not the general recommendation on levels of cholesterol is applicable to everyone. I am not sure that it really is. I say that because I see people with high cholesterol levels in their 70s and 80s who clearly have no coronary artery disease. We also see young people in their 20s and 30s with low cholesterol who have very severe coronary artery disease. So, there is a subset of people who have a predisposition to coronary artery disease who will benefit from a prudent diet and a lower level of cholesterol. For others, who do not have a predisposition to coronary artery disease, it may really not matter.

4. *Two types of cholesterol are described in the literature: the "good" high density lipoproteins (HDLs) and the "bad" low density lipoproteins (LDLs). If a person maintains a level of cholesterol below 200, does he or she have to be concerned about the ratio of high to low density lipoproteins?*

The HDLs are those which tend to carry cholesterol into the liver and out of the body. The higher the level of HDLs, the more cholesterol can be moved out of the body. The LDLs are those which tend to accumulate in the heart and the blood vessels.

People who have total levels of cholesterol under 200 generally have a normal or high HDL level and a low LDL level. Some people, however, who have a cholesterol of 200 or under have a very low HDL cholesterol and an elevated LDL level. This is unusual. When we screen a patient and find a total cholesterol level of 150 to 170, it is generally inappropriate to look for HDL or LDL. However, I might look for those two lipoproteins if the individual has a bad family history. If the total cholesterol level is above 200, then the levels of HDLs and LDLs should be checked.

5. *What is the ideal ratio of HDLs to LDLs?*

The HDL should be over 55 and the LDL should be under 130 to 150. No one is absolutely certain what the best number is. This also varies with the methods of biochemical testing, which vary from laboratory to laboratory. As a result of the differences, the normal levels vary from laboratory to laboratory. Consequently, the general guide of maintaining cholesterol under 200 may not be applicable to every laboratory report. For some laboratories, any reported level under 240 might be acceptable, since their cholesterol determination includes other elements in the blood which test similar to cholesterol. You have to know what your laboratory's normal values are. This information is provided to your doctor.

6. *"Finger prick" tests to measure cholesterol are now being offered. Would you comment on these?*

They may not be very accurate and result either in undue anxiety or undue assurance that all is well.

7. *If you have a high level of cholesterol, what kind of a diet would you recommend?*

I provide some very simple guidelines. Don't eat any eggs or meat. Just eat fish and fowl, and drink skim milk—not whole milk. Never eat ice cream or ice milk, eat sherbet. Don't put cream in your coffee, use skim milk. Don't eat cheese, even low-fat cheese. If you follow these guidelines, you will generally be on a low-fat diet.

8. *Is caffeine harmful?*

It is thought that caffeine may raise the level of harmful LDLs in the blood. The major problem with excessive caffeine is an increase in heart rate. If your heart is normal, it really doesn't matter. If you have any evidence of heart disease, you don't want to race the heart; therefore you should not take caffeine.

For the normal person, one or two cups of caffeinated coffee a day is certainly alright. There is no evidence that caffeine enhances the development of coronary artery disease. On the other hand, if coronary artery disease is suspected, I tell patients not to drink caffeinated coffee.

9. *What is the importance of triglycerides to heart disease?*

It used to be thought that they were very important. Probably they are not. The importance of triglycerides is mainly that they may be a marker for diabetes. They are much, much less important than cholesterol as a factor in coronary heart disease.

10. *Recently, some doctors have recommended taking small doses of aspirin regularly to reduce the chance of heart disease. Do you support the recommendation?*

Taking aspirin to reduce the chances of contracting heart disease is a popular misconception. The physicians that did the study did not say that at all. A recent study on aspirin and heart disease indicates that if you have had a heart attack, the administration of aspirin reduces the possibility of a second heart attack. There is also some evidence that if you are having a heart attack, and get to a hospital very quickly, the use of a thrombolytic agent such as streptokinase or TPA, along with aspirin, will open your arteries more effectively than if aspirin is not used with one of these agents.

There is no evidence that aspirin will prevent coronary heart disease. It would be nice if that were true. Then, you could start children on one aspirin every day or every other day and prevent coronary heart disease. But nobody has ever conducted such a study.

We cannot say that aspirin reduces the chances of heart disease, because "heart disease" is much too global a statement. Aspirin does not have any effect on hypertensive heart disease, valvular heart disease, or myocardial heart disease. The only effect aspirin has is on coronary heart disease, and, more specifically, on the coronary heart disease that occurs after a heart attack. *There is no evidence that long-term taking of aspirin will prevent you from having a first heart attack or will prevent you from ultimately ending up with coronary artery disease.*

11. *How important is a high fiber diet in cancer avoidance?*

Probably important in preventing colon cancer and breast cancer. There is no evidence that it prevents any other type of cancer. Based on population studies, it appears that eating a high fiber diet reduces the incidence of colon and breast cancer. There also seems to be some evidence that if you eat a low fat diet, you reduce your risk of cancer. Other studies suggest that high fat diets increase the risk of cancer. The fact is that we don't know the relationship between diet and the development of cancer.

It may be that much of the cancer we see associated with various kinds of diets is really associated with the preservative additives rather than the food itself.

12. *Are you suggesting that some preservatives cause cancer?*

It may be. No one knows what causes cancer.

13. *Fish oil supplements are advertised as being helpful in reducing the level of blood cholesterol. Please comment.*

It certainly has made some people rich. There is no evidence that fish oil supplements have done very much to reduce cholesterol. The link between fish oil and cholesterol is based on the fact that Eskimos eat a very high—80 percent—fat diet. Their incidence of coronary heart disease is low. They eat a lot of fish, which accounts for the oils in their diet. An ad-hoc kind of reasoning suggests that if Eskimos eat a lot of fish, and fish have a lot of fish oils, and Eskimos have a low incidence of coronary disease, then you will lower your cholesterol and consequently have a lower incidence of coronary artery disease if you eat fish oils.

We find very few scientific studies looking at this question. *There have been a few very preliminary studies which suggest that high quantities of these fish oils may actually accelerate coronary artery disease.* What I recommend to my patients is simply, don't waste your time taking fish oils. Eat lots of fish, as the Eskimos do. But don't take *concentrated* amounts of fish oils. These large doses may also have an adverse effect on calcium metabolism. *Clearly, fish oils in capsule form are to be avoided, in my opinion.*

14. *How does a person know what their "optimum" weight should be, given their height, age, and body build?*

Insurance company data was collected to suggest the best height to weight ratios. It may be that a person's ideal weight may be too low or too high. It depends so much on other factors.

Let's say an individual is tall and very thin (15 to 20 pounds under what his or her "ideal" weight should be), and his or her cholesterol is normal or low, blood pressure is normal, and he or she doesn't smoke. What difference does it make if he or she is underweight? Let's say a person is free of all those risk factors and is overweight by 15 to 20 pounds. That really doesn't matter.

We have very little evidence on what it means to be underweight. Some "soft" studies indicate that being underweight increases the chances of dying from infectious diseases and some types of cancer, but the evidence is very questionable.

15. *Does that mean that being underweight causes some of these diseases?*

We don't know. Cause and effect in all of this material is unknown. The reason is that we don't know what causes coronary artery disease. We don't know what causes cancer. We do know that if you have certain attributes, you are more likely to have coronary heart disease or cancer.

If you are 20% above the statistical "ideal" weight for your height and age, you are more likely to have elevated cholesterol, have high blood pressure, be a smoker, and be diabetic, all of which has an adverse affect on the development of coronary artery disease.

Another example is cancer of the lungs. *It is clear that if you are a cigarette smoker, you are more likely to contract cancer of the lung than if you are a nonsmoker.* But there are people who smoke two packs a day and do not contract lung cancer. Can we say, therefore, that there is a direct cause and effect link between smoking and contracting lung cancer? Probably so. But it is likely that an intermediary process is at work within the biochemistry and the genetics of the person that comes between the offending agent (smoking) and the development of the disease (lung cancer).

16. *How important is it that a person maintain his/her "optimum" body weight?*

I think it is important to maintain your optimum weight because you are less likely to have associated risk factors for coronary artery disease.

17. *Does the incidence of coronary heart disease vary as a function of weight change?*

A mythology has arisen which says that going on a very spartan diet, such as the Pritikin diet, and losing a great deal of weight, will result in the dissolving or removing of plaques from the coronary arteries. Unfortunately, no one has ever proven that. There is no evidence that losing weight and reducing your level of cholesterol from even 300 to 100 will make plaques in your arteries disappear. The loss of weight and the reduction of cholesterol may prevent or slow down the development of coronary artery disease, but there is no evidence that it will remove the plaques that already exist in the blood vessels.

18. *Is there any way through diet or medication to remove the cholesterol in the blood vessels?*

We don't have coronary artery "Drano" yet. Someday, I am sure there will be a chemical that can be inserted directly into the arteries to dissolve those terrible plaques.

19. *Some people weigh less than their "optimum" weight. Does being "underweight" add to the incidence of heart disease?*

Certainly it does not, because if your weight is lower than optimum, your heart does not have to work as hard and you are less likely to have risk factors for coronary heart disease.

STRESS AND "TYPE A" BEHAVIOR

The finest art, the most
difficult to learn, is the art
of living.
John Macy

1. *Stress has been identified as an important factor in causing coronary heart disease. From a medical viewpoint, what is stress?*

I am not certain what role stress plays in coronary heart disease. It is clear that when you are under stress, your level of adrenalin and adrenocortical hormones increases. Both of these tend to accelerate the development of coronary heart disease. It is also possible that stress, through these agents, causes spasm in the coronary arteries. Spasm causes injury to the vessel walls, and this is where cholesterol can become lodged. But, the evidence of this process is very soft.

Stress, therefore, probably does play a role in the development of coronary disease. It may play a more significant role in worsening already existing coronary disease. For example, when you are really under stress and your body produces corticosteroids and adrenalin, it makes your blood thicker. If you already have plaques, it may precipitate the development of a clot in a coronary artery, or perhaps a stroke. But, the role of stress is not very well defined. In terms of being a risk factor, it is not in the same league as smoking, high blood pressure or a significantly elevated cholesterol.

Stress may play a role in high blood pressure. It is clear that stress will increase blood pressure.

Stress can be positive. The individual who loves his or her job and is under normal job stress and pressure is not in an adverse situation. But consider the stress resulting from the death of a close family member. That is highly negative stress. People indeed do tend to have coronary events around a tragedy such as that.

2. *It has been argued that people have always been under stress. Do you think that stress is increasing for most people or have we just become more attuned to the concept of stress*

I think the level of stress is increasing in our society. There is no question about that. The stresses of a modern, high-technology society are undoubtedly different from those found in a primitive society. The society in which we live, with the breakdown of the family unit, the fast pace at which we work—all have increased stress. I think that with the increase in stress, people have become more cognizant of it and have tried various methods to reduce it. Whether reduction of stress will materially reduce coronary artery heart disease is questionable. I am not sure it will.

3. *As a cardiologist, what have you found to be most effective in controlling stress for your patients?*

There are two types of stress. First, consider the successful individual who is under a lot of stress on his or her job. It is not my job as a cardiologist to suggest that he or she resign and go sleep on the beach. I can't do that. The stress is there, and the individual must face it and deal with it. There are millions of people in this situation.

Second, there are the personal stresses in one's life. From a cardiologist's viewpoint, there are possibilities of mitigating that stress by talking with the patient's spouse or other significant family members. If the stress is inordinate and difficult, I try to get my patients into the hands of a psychologist or psychiatrist who is more capable of dealing with the problem.

4. *Do you feel that people who exhibit "Type A" behavior are more prone to heart disease?*

They certainly are not more prone to most types of heart disease. It has been said that they are more prone to coronary heart disease and high blood pressure, however. There may be a little truth to that. But the fact is, we see a lot of "Type B" people with heart disease and a lot of "Type A" people who don't have it.

What is "Type A" behavior? Probably the answer is the person who is constantly making deadlines. You can be a "Type A" person who doesn't smoke, who doesn't have high blood pressure or elevated cholesterol, and is prudent with diet. But "Type A" individuals tend to be smokers, tend to eat too much, and exercise infrequently. They therefore tend to have the risk factors that increase the probability of coronary artery disease. *As in the case with being overweight, "Type A" behavior is a marker of those individuals who are more likely to have those other risk factors.* The "Type A" behavior in itself is probably not a risk factor.

PREPARING CHILDREN FOR GOOD HEALTH

Children are our most
valuable natural resource.
Herbert Hoover

1. *How old should a person be before he or she starts to become concerned about heart disease?*

Again, it is a matter of which type of heart disease. For example, there is little you can do about valvular heart disease. You are either born with it or you acquire it by having rheumatic fever. If you have congenital heart disease, you were born with it, and it should be detected and treated appropriately.

You should be conscious of three types of heart disease: hypertensive heart disease, coronary heart disease and dilated cardiomyopathies. Let's consider the dilated cardiomyopathies first because these are the easiest to discuss. There is no question that in our society, alcohol is the most likely cause of this condition, which is characterized by a flabby heart muscle that doesn't contract well. Therefore, *moderation in alcohol should start at a very young age.*

Next, let's consider hypertensive heart disease. Again, so much depends upon family history and a reasonably early physical exam. A person in his or her 20s should have a blood pressure check and, perhaps, a cardiogram for use as a baseline. As for high blood pressure, which tends to run in families, there's not much evidence that a person without such a family history needs to be too concerned. High blood pressure is associated with heart failure and stroke. The only way to know if you have high blood pressure is to have it taken at regular intervals. This is probably one of the best things about going for a regular physical exam.

Coronary heart disease is the most difficult to discuss, because the question is, should avoidance start in childhood? For example, should you regulate your children's diets to avoid the development of coronary heart disease?

It is hard to say whether or not we should severely restrict the ingestion of milk, eggs, and ice cream in children. But, *parents should get their children to avoid the junk foods, the fast-food hamburgers, the cheeseburgers which are just loaded with fats and additives.* A great deal of preventive heart disease can start in the home with the development of a prudent diet in childhood. What you learn to eat as a child will be very important in determining what you eat as an adult. *Certainly, one of the best things parents can do for their children is not to smoke. It is the worst risk factor and should be inculcated into the child that he or she should not smoke. Also, since passive smoking (i.e. being in the presence of someone who is smoking) is almost as harmful as smoking, parents who smoke in the presence of their children are putting them at risk. As a risk prevention method, I would be sure that my children are not smokers.*

Once you are in your 20s and 30s, the most rational thing to do is look at your mother and father. If they are in their 80s, are hale and hearty, never had a heart attack, are not diabetic, and don't have high blood pressure, the chances that you will have such problems is pretty small. It is still worthwhile to have your blood pressure checked, have a cardiogram, have your blood sugar tested, and your blood fats checked every four or five years.

On the other hand, suppose you have a bad family history. I would suggest that you have a very careful screen of cholesterol, triglycerides, HDLs, LDLs, blood sugar, blood pressure, a baseline rest cardiogram, and even an exercise cardiogram every other year when you are in your 20s. Beyond 30 or 35, these tests should be done yearly. If everything stays normal, that's fine. If any abnormality is detected, it should be appropriately treated.

So much depends on family history and what a person picks up from that family history. In some instances, it is difficult to predict heart disease because we just don't know what causes coronary artery disease. For example, one of the most tragic cases I have seen involved a young person with terrible coronary heart disease, which was not anticipated because there was no family history of the disease. If a family history of the disease had existed, avoidance measures might have been taken.

You have to look at things from a statistical viewpoint. If you have a good family history, the chances of your having significant coronary heart disease or significant high blood pressure are pretty small.

The importance of educating people to family history is very important. The American Heart Association has played an important role in the education of people. Nowhere can education be more important than in getting people to alter their lifestyles if they have a predisposition to coronary heart disease or high blood pressure.

Company Index

Subject Index